S0-BMY-484

LIBRARY
LENOIR RHYNE COLLEGE

WITHDRAWN

WITHDRAWN

BIOLOGY AND SOCIETY

THE EVOLUTION OF MAN AND HIS TECHNOLOGY

BIOLOGY AND

Under the general editorship of
NORMAN H. GILES and RICHARD A. GOLDSBY

SOCIETY

THE EVOLUTION OF MAN AND HIS TECHNOLOGY

ANDREW McCLARY   Michigan State University

MACMILLAN PUBLISHING CO., INC.
New York

COLLIER MACMILLAN PUBLISHERS
London

CARL A. RUDISILL LIBRARY
LENOIR RHYNE COLLEGE

301.31
M13b
96018
Feb. 1976

Copyright © 1975, Andrew McClary
Printed in the United States of America

All rights reserved. No part of this book may be reproduced or
transmitted in any form or by any means, electronic or mechanical,
including photocopying, recording, or any information storage and
retrieval system, without permission in writing from the Publisher.

Macmillan Publishing Co., Inc.
866 Third Avenue, New York, New York 10022
Collier-Macmillan Canada, Ltd.

Library of Congress Cataloging in Publication Data

McClary, Andrew.
  Biology and society.

  Bibliography: p.
  1. Human ecology.   2. Technology—History.
3. Hygiene.   I.   Title.   [DNLM: 1. Civilization.
2. Environment.   3. Evolution.   4. Technology.
CB478 M126b]
GF47.M28   301.31   73–20994
ISBN 0–02–378510–1

Printing: 1 2 3 4 5 6 7 8   Year: 5 6 7 8 9 0

To Ann and Susan

PREFACE

This book was written with one aim in mind: to argue that we can make more sense out of the thorny problems facing our technological society if we view them from an evolutionary perspective.

Rather than present the reader with an encyclopedic mass of information, I have tried instead to focus on these questions: How and why has our technological society evolved? What are its key characteristics? In what ways can we direct its further evolution in order to create the best of possible future societies? It is my hope that readers from diverse fields may find the views developed in the book interesting or controversial enough to merit further investigation.

I would like to thank David Armstrong, University of Colorado; Arthur Borror, University of New Hampshire; Norman Giles, University of Georgia; Jerry Wilhm, Oklahoma State University; and Manfred Englemann, Robert McDaniel, John Mullins, and Marvin Solomon, all of Michigan State University, who read the manuscript and made many helpful suggestions. Hurd Hutchins and Charles Stewart of Macmillan have been of great aid in the preparation of the book, and I feel particularly indebted to Peter Loewer who did the illustrations. My wife, Jane, has made many helpful suggestions and has typed the entire manuscript. Finally, I would like to thank all the students who have challenged me to try to make some sense of modern technology.

A. McC.

_____CONTENTS

The last living remnants of primitive man are disappearing from the earth. A very few groups, such as the recently discovered Tasaday of the Philippines, are still virtually untouched by the modern world. Others, such as the Bushmen, are either dying out or are in the process of transition to Western culture.

Is this change inevitable, and if so, does it represent progress? Until twenty or thirty years ago doubters were few, but now a rising voice of disillusionment and dismay is heard.

In his recent book *Overskill* Eugene Schwartz puts it this way:

mindless technology is inundating the world, sweeping all before it. Although the graphs of "progress" continue to rise, man is only now beginning to perceive the price that is exacted to enable the fountains of technology to continue to spew forth their promise. Mingled with the "Eureka" cries that accompany the scaling of new heights of scientific achievement are the rising wails of mankind who suffer from these same achievements. . . . We have sowed our fields with trisodium phosphate and there are more hungry people in the world than ever before. We have built hospitals and clinics and there are more sick people than ever before. We have built schools and illiteracy flourishes. We have built factories and filled them with machines and find that we are slaves to the machines.[1]

And yet, as Philip Handler, president of the National Academy of Sciences, recently said:

> Those who reject science charge that, through technology, science has engendered our environmental problems, degraded the quality of life, limited our personal freedom, and has been the willing servant of the military. Each is perhaps a partial truth. Yet the fact remains that there is no tool but additional science-based technology, appropriately regulated by an understanding society, with which yet further to improve the human condition. . . . I deny that my life has been made wretched or my freedom reduced by science. Rather do I believe that technology has made the lives of about three-quarters of all Americans richer, more comfortable, more enjoyable, and more healthy, than that of humanity in any other period of history.[2]

How do we really fare? Is mankind better off under modern science and technology? Or is it a matter of trade offs—a gain in some ways under Western culture and a loss in others? How can we decide?

We propose to examine these questions in an evolutionary context. We shall begin our inquiry by a look at that unique organization of matter called life. Next, we will turn to the evolution of modern man and his culture.

Finally, we will return to the question just raised: Is modern man's life a better one than that of his ancestors?

PAST

PART I

1
LIFE

What is it that characterizes a living thing and makes it somehow different from an inanimate object, such as a rock? Each biology textbook seems to have its own list of life's characteristics, which may suggest that we have asked an unanswerable question. Perhaps a more reasonable question would be: What are some of the important characteristics of life? We offer four characteristics as crucial to being alive: integration, reproduction, homeostasis, and energy capture. To illustrate them, let's look at hydra, a small fresh-water animal.

HYDRA

1. *General characteristics.* Hydras are found in fresh-water ponds, lakes, and streams throughout the world. Although common, they are easily overlooked because they are so small. A careful examination of vegetation, boards, rocks, or other material taken from a pond will reveal what appear to be groups of small, frazzled threads growing from the collected material. Upon magnification, each thread becomes an individual animal consisting of an elongated, cylindrical body topped by a circlet of tentacles (Figure 1-1). At the center of the tentacles is an opening which leads into a simple internal digestive cavity. A hydra will normally measure around one-eighth inch in length. To talk about length, however, reflects the human bias that

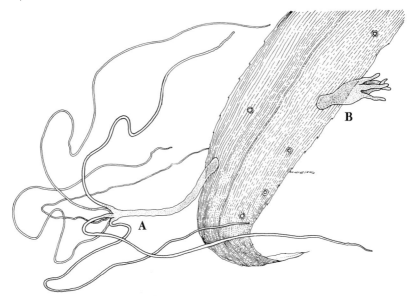

Figure 1-1. A. Hydra in a relaxed state. B. Hydra in a contracted state.

all organisms resemble man in having fixed dimensions. Hydra is much more versatile than this and has a remarkable capacity to alter its size and shape.

2. *Integration.* Hydra is an organized entity composed of many cells, each of which cooperates with, and is dependent upon, its neighbors. Each kind of cell has its own particular jobs to do. Certain cells on the tentacles, for example, are specialized to capture prey. These cells contain stinging capsules called *nematocysts. Penetrant nematocysts* spear their victims and inject a paralyzing poison. *Volvent nemato-cysts* help to entangle the prey (Figure 1-2). Hungry hydras are usually quite active and bend in all directions, which increases the chance of their tentacles contacting food. A small animal which hap-pens to hit a tentacle will be immobilized by nematocysts and then carried toward the hydra's mouth, which opens even before the food has arrived. Feeding or other movements are coordinated by special sensory cells and by contractile cells which cause the hydra's body to change its shape or position.

After it has been ingested, hydra's food is partially broken down by enzymes in the digestive cavity. These are released by special gland cells. Other cells have hairlike flagella which whip about, circulating food through the cavity. Contractions of hydra's body also help this circulation. After the food is thoroughly broken up and circulated, digestive cells lining the cavity will absorb it. These cells extend finger-like *pseudopods,* which engulf the food and carry it into their protoplasm. The digestive cells then pass the ingested food along to other cells in hydra's body.

In addition to food, oxygen is also taken into hydra's cells. No specialized cells are necessary for this in an animal the size of hydra. Oxygen simply passes across the body wall and into the cells which line it.

The food and oxygen thus obtained are utilized by cells primarily to produce energy, secondarily to produce needed cell materials.

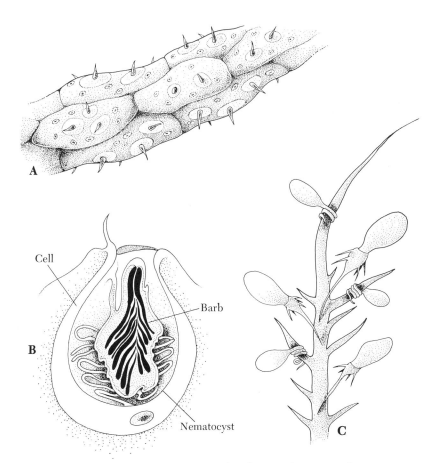

Figure 1-2. A. Portion of hydra's tentacle, showing batteries of nematocysts. B. Undischarged penetrant nematocyst. C. Discharged penetrant and volvent nematocysts on a bristle of a crustacean. (All after Barnes, Robert D., *Invertebrate Zoology,* Philadelphia: W.B. Saunders Company, 1968).

As an integrate, hydra is completely dependent on the function of all those cells of which it is composed. Without their specialized abilities, it ceases to be hydra. In turn, the individual cells have no meaning apart from the animal they form. There are no individualists or prima donnas among the cells of hydra.

Many inanimate things are made up of units. Unlike cells, however, the units of non-living things are largely independent aggregates rather than interdependent integrates. Furthermore, removing some of these units will do little, if anything, to change the character of the object to which they belong. A sandpile, for example, is not an integrated thing, but an aggregate composed of millions of essentially independent grains. Removing one shovelful will decrease the size of the pile a bit but will not alter its fundamental characteristics.

3. *Reproduction.* In hydra, reproduction can be either asexual or sexual. In asexual reproduction, which usually takes place during warmer months, a bud appears on the side of a mature individual. It begins as a bulge, grows into a stalk, develops tentacles, and eventually detaches from the parent as a new hydra. Sexual reproduction usually takes place in the fall. Some species of hydra are *dioecious;* that is, any one hydra is either a male and produces sperm, or a female and produces eggs. Other species, however, are *monoecious;* that is, one individual produces both eggs and sperm. The many sperm are produced within a testis located on the upper half of the body wall. Ovaries, which are usually located lower on the body wall, each produce a single egg (Figure 1-3). Sperm escape through a nipple on the testis and swim about. Several sperm may penetrate one ovary, but only one enters the egg itself. After fertilization, an egg will transform into an embryo which is covered with a resistant shell. The embryo will then either drop off or be placed on the substrate through bending movements of its parent. After a period of dormancy which may last over the winter, the shell breaks and a young hydra develops from the cell mass inside.

We take reproduction for granted and rarely think of how unique a process it is. Only life can create such specialized objects as sperm, eggs, or buds and then transform them into an adult of the species.

4. *Homeostasis.* Homeostasis is the tendency of living things to maintain a normative or usual form and to return to that form after some event has distorted it. Hydra's remarkable ability to regenerate lost or damaged parts is a form of homeostatic activity. If its tentacles are removed, they will rapidly regrow. If a hydra is cut into several pieces,

each will regenerate into a completely new animal. It is possible to take a portion of hydra's body and mash it into a small globe of disorganized tissue, and, if conditions are favorable, the globe will regenerate into a new hydra (Figure 1-4). If one is careful, it is even possible to turn a hydra inside-out. The animal will then respond by exchanging its inner and outer body walls so that they are once again positioned normally.

Homeostasis is a unique property of life. It is true that some inanimate objects have a kind of pseudo-homeostasis. A drop of mercury, for example, will return to a spherical shape after distortion, and certain dissolved salts will repeatedly form one kind of crystal when evaporated. In living things, however, homeostatic activity is far more sophisticated, for it involves the maintenance of an integrate rather than an aggregate.

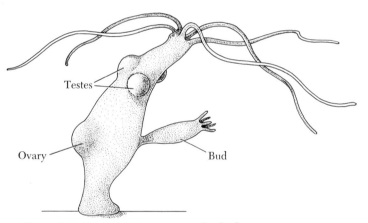

Figure 1-3. Reproductive organs of a hydra.

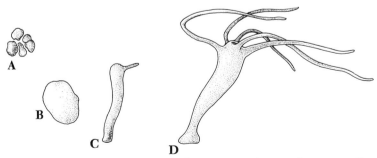

Figure 1-4. Regeneration in a hydra. A. Bits of tissue form; B. a flat sac; C. a cylinder; D. a reformed hydra.

5. *Energy capture.* Because it is an aggregate, a sandpile is easily dispersed. It will not fight the shovel which seeks to destroy it. In contrast, living things not only resist disruption, they go further and seek to increase their own kind. This does not necessarily mean they consciously strive to do this, but merely that it is in the nature of life to build more of itself. If life has any one overriding characteristic, it is the stubborn struggle it wages against *entropy*. The term entropy refers to the tendency of matter and energy to become dispersed in a random, disorganized fashion through the cosmos. In building more of their own kind, living things such as hydra fight this trend.

A large part of hydra's behavior, particularly that which we call feeding, is directed toward capturing the energy and matter needed

ENTROPY

Most astronomers believe that the universe began about ten billion years ago in the form of a primordial fireball or *ylem*. This primordial mass contained all the matter of the universe, condensed at a temperature of millions of degrees and at an incredible density of over 100 million tons per cubic centimeter. The ylem-matter first consisted of free sub-atomic particles. The universe was created through an explosion of this primordial fireball. As the fireball expanded, its temperature and pressure dropped, and primordial atoms began to form. Calculations indicate that all of the ninety-two natural elements appeared within a half hour. Continued expansion, cooling, and condensation of matter then produced the universe in which we now live. The evolution of our universe, which began with the primordial fireball, is still under way. Not only do its stars and galaxies continue to race away from each other, but a second and more fundamental trend continues. This is a trend toward a state of complete entropy in the universe.

Roughly speaking, the word entropy means disorganization. Should we ever reach a state of complete entropy, matter and energy will be evenly dispersed everywhere, all integration of matter will be lost, and the dark universe will consist of endlessly drifting, lifeless matter. At first thought, it might seem that living things have risen above the entropy problem, but this is not the case, for the following reasons.

All work is accomplished through molecular motion, or energy. This work-energy has a basic trait: it can never flow uphill. To illustrate this, imagine a group of people gathered about a fire. The

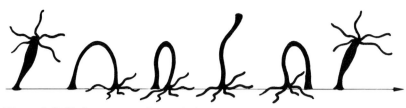

Figure 1-5. Hydra somersaulting. (After Wagner, as given in Hegner, Robert W., *Invertebrate Zoology*. New York: Macmillan Publishing Co., Inc., 1933.)

to maintain its organization and integrity and to build more of its own kind. When hungry, for example, hydra will elongate to an inch or more and sweep its tentacles about, seeking food. If food becomes too scarce, hydra can move to a new location by gliding, somersaulting, or

heat energy of the burning wood is diffused outward into the molecules of the air and to those molecules which compose the people surrounding the fire. That is, the high heat energy of the fire tends to spread out into surrounding objects, to flow downhill from a hot or high-energy area to cooler, lower-energy ones. But the opposite of this, a flow of dispersed heat into cold logs until they burst into flame, never occurs spontaneously. It can be done by conscious work effort; for example, man can devise some machine to accomplish it. Yet the work of this machine, or any other kind of work we know of, is never completely efficient. No matter how hard we try, we will find that either some of the energy our machine tries to capture will escape its attentions or that the machine itself will be dispersing some of its own work energy into the surrounding environment. This same wasting of energy occurs among all living things. In carrying out our daily work, we are never one hundred per cent efficient—we always burn more energy than we actually use. Thus, entropy, the obstinate tendency for matter and energy to spread out into even distribution in the environment, seems a characteristic of both the living and nonliving.

Is there no way to avoid entropy? If there is, it will probably be found in that human product of evolution we call culture. For it is basic to the character of life, and of man in particular, to wage an endless war on entropy. Perhaps, as one writer has commented, life may yet succeed against all odds in molding the universe to its own purposes.

rising to the surface on a gas bubble produced by its foot (Figure 1-5). If starved and then presented with macerated food, hydra will literally turn itself inside out in an attempt to reach the food.

In our effort to understand life we have been concentrating on the characteristics of individual organisms. We now wish to change our focus a bit and look at groups of organisms. Not all organisms belong to groups such as families or societies, but all must belong to an ecosystem.

A POND ECOSYSTEM

A typical fresh-water pond contains hundreds of different species of plants and animals. Some of these, such as the rooted plants or larger fish, are quite conspicuous. Others, such as the various species of hydra or the many microscopic protozoa, would only be noticed by a biologist. Superficially, a pond seems a chaotic jumble of competing organisms. On more careful examination, however, one comes to realize that order exists within the pond, for it contains an interdependent community of plants and animals. This community, together with the environment it occupies, is called an *ecosystem*. All ecosystems have certain characteristics:

1. *An ecosystem receives its energy from the sun.* If we examine the plants within the pond, we find that all have one thing in common. Through photosynthesis they convert the light energy which they receive from the sun into chemical energy, which is bound into sugar molecules. This sugar can be used to build other kinds of molecules or it can be burnt to provide the plants with work energy. Using this sugar and the minerals available in the pond, the plants build more of their own kind.

2. *The flow of matter in an ecosystem is cyclic.* Collectively, the pond's plants are called *producers*. The plants provide food for a second group of pond dwellers, the *primary consumers*. These are usually small animals, such as water fleas. The primary consumers, in turn, are eaten by *secondary consumers*. Although hydra is one of the latter, many secondary consumers are animals larger than hydra, such as fish. *Decomposers* then continue the cycle by attacking the wastes formed by producers or consumers and converting it into the minerals which are once again used by producer plants.

Some of the organic and inorganic matter cycling from producer to consumer to decomposer is lost from the pond, but the bulk of it moves

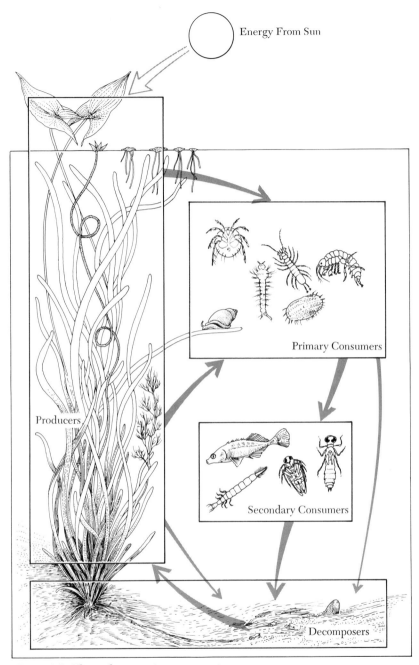

Figure 1-6. Flow of matter in an ecosystem.

Energy From Sun

Producers

Primary Consumers

Secondary Consumers

Decomposers

endlessly through the cycle. Sometimes this matter short circuits, skipping some stage in the cycle. For example, most of the dead leaves

13

and stems of water plants will go directly to decomposers rather than to consumers. Because of this, a hundred pounds of producer plants might support ten pounds of primary consumers and these in turn support only four pounds of secondary consumers. Figure 1-6 depicts the ecosystem cycle we have described.

3. *The flow of matter in an ecosystem is actually very complex.* The ecosystem cycle which we have been describing is a generalization,

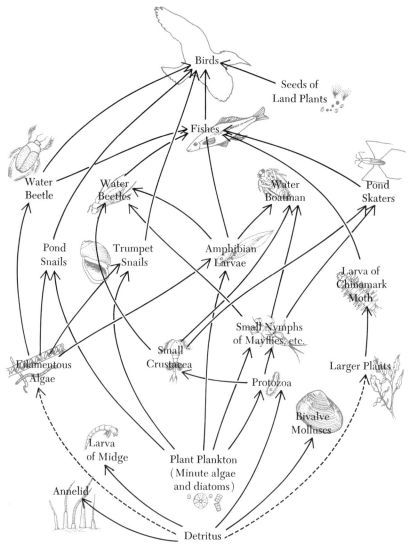

Figure 1-7. Some food pathways in a pond ecosystem.

an abstraction which tells us what happens to the matter within the pond over long periods of time. Should we examine the pond at one point in time, we receive a quite different impression. Then, the pond's matter would seem to flow through a series of very complicated pathways (Figure 1-7).

All living things belong to ecosystems. Some ecosystems are large, some small; some have many member species, some few. All, however, have cycles of the kind described above. If we compare an ecosystem with an individual organism such as hydra, some interesting similarities appear. First, both organism and ecosystem are integrates. Just as was true for the cells of hydra, the various species within an ecosystem cannot exist in isolation. Second, both organism and ecosystem tend to be homeostatic. When disrupted, an organism will either die or regenerate to its normal form. When disrupted, an ecosystem will tend to do the same. In the case of ecosystems, however, the regeneration process differs somewhat. Stable or *mature* ecosystems are characterized by complexity. That is, they contain many species and have many food pathways. Disrupted ecosystems, such as might occur from flooding or as a result of man's activities, are typically much simplified in the number of species and food pathways they contain. Regeneration toward the norm thus implies a long period of change, or, as an ecologist would put it, *succession* toward a condition of stable complexity. Finally, both organism and ecosystem are energy-capturing machines. Both counterbalance entropy by taking energy from outside. Both distribute it among their constituent members in order to build more of their own kind.

WHAT IS THE DRIVING FORCE BEHIND LIFE?

Living things are integrated, reproducing, homeostatic, energy-capturing systems.

To some people, these characteristics mean that life can only be explained by assuming the presence of some *vital life force* which is resident in living tissues and is beyond the power of rational science to explain. The late Edmund Sinnott, a well-known vitalist, put it this way:

Matter is not master. If in the universe there is an organizing principle, it may be that some of it dwells in each of us as his own soul—not as a transient and temporary configuration in atoms and molecules and quanta, but part of an eternal, universal spirit. . . .[3]

Most biologists oppose vitalism. Many are *mechanists* and would agree with this statement by Dean Wooldridge, author of the book *Mechanical Man:*

> we seem justified in the broadest possible application of what may be called the central thesis of physical biology: that a single body of natural laws operating on a single set of material particles completely accounts for the origin and properties of living organisms as well as nonliving aggregations of matter and man-made structures. Accordingly, man is essentially no more than a complex machine.[4]

Wooldridge's concept of life is also *reductionistic.* That is, it assumes that all of life's properties reside in the units of which a living thing is made. In effect, it says one could dissect a hydra into its constitutent cells or atoms, learn the characteristics of these, and from this information understand what a hydra is. To many mechanistic biologists the key unit of life is neither atom nor cell, but *DNA. Genes,* built of DNA, guide all homeostatic activity, for they code the information as to what is normal for any one kind of life. DNA also directs and coordinates cell activity and thus accounts for the integrative and energy-capturing characteristics of living things. To a mechanist, then, living things, whether hydras or people, are complex machines. The difference between a life machine and another kind of machine lies not in some mysterious quality of the former, but in the particular way its units are organized and directed.

Many biologists agree with the mechanists in their emphasis on DNA's importance but maintain that the mechanistic explanation is not sufficient to account for the properties of life. The mechanist tends to view living things as if they existed in isolation, but many biologists argue that life can only be understood *holistically* as part of a much larger system. In order to understand a hydra, one needs to understand its environment, for the form and behavior of a hydra is strongly conditioned by the environment in which it lives. Some holists enlarge their argument to include inanimate things as well. Michael Polanyi, for example, argues that no object or entity can be understood except as a part of a larger whole. Since our senses are finite, but the larger whole is infinite, the implication is that we must be forever limited in our attempts to understand the meaning of life.

These views are discussed and defended in a number of interesting and readable paperbacks; a few are listed in the bibliography at the end of this book.

2 _____LIFE AND EVOLUTION

ADAPTATION

One of the most intriguing things about plants and animals is the way in which they seem to fit their environments. Each species seems carefully designed or adapted to meet the particular demands of its environment. To illustrate this, we will look at two environments, a rocky shore and man himself.

Life on a Rocky Shore

Rocky shores, such as one finds along the New England coast, are highly demanding environments. Unprotected plants or animals can be pounded to death by the waves. Food is available, but specialized techniques are needed to harvest it. The shifting tides force organisms on a rocky shore to spend part of their time submerged and part exposed.

A number of plants and animals have developed adaptations to surmount these challenges. Barnacles (Figure 2-1A) are among the most common rocky shore animals. The barnacle's tentlike shell is glued firmly to the rock and is constructed of movable plates so that the shell can be opened when the animal feeds but closed when the tide is out or when the waves are excessively strong. The barnacle itself lives in an upside-down position in the shell. It feeds by extending

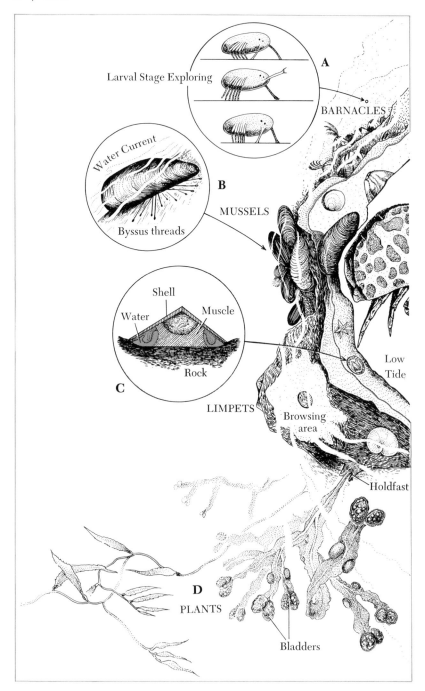

Larval Stage Exploring

A

BARNACLES

Water Current

B

Byssus threads

MUSSELS

Shell

Water

Muscle

Rock

C

LIMPETS

Low
Tide

Browsing
area

Holdfast

D

PLANTS

Bladders

Figure 2-1. Some adaptations to a rocky shore. See text for details.

its feet from the shell and capturing bits of food from the surrounding water. Sensory receptors of the kind found on more active animals are absent. Young barnacles are free-swimming for a brief period, then settle and attach themselves to rock surfaces. Once attached, a barnacle is committed for life to its choice of habitat. Before attaching itself, a barnacle will land and test various surfaces until an ideal spot is found.

Mussels (Figure 2-1B), which also are common on rocky shores, are attached to the rocks by tough *byssus* threads. These serve to anchor each mussel, yet leave enough play so that the mussel can swing with the current. The mussel shell is streamlined, which minimizes wave impact. Its byssus threads are attached in such a way that the mussel tends to swing with its narrow end facing into the sea. At low tide the mussel's shell closes tightly to protect the animal from dessication. Mussels are similar to barnacles in that they feed by straining particulate food from sea water. Also, as is the case with barnacles, mussels' sensory organs are reduced or absent.

The limpet (Figure 2-1C) is another common rocky shore dweller. A limpet's shell has a low profile, which provides the least possible resistance to wave action, and its foot is flattened out to provide maximum holding power against waves and currents. When feeding, a limpet moves slowly along, feeding on the algae which cover the rock. Each limpet has a home base located approximately in the center of its browsing range, consisting of a shallow depression, worn by many visits and shaped for a watertight fit with the limpet's shell. This ingenious adaptation allows the limpet, during periods of low tide, to remain bathed in the water that is trapped inside its shell.

Many rocky shore plants (Figure 2-1D) have *holdfasts*, or organs of attachment, which are extremely strong. Usually, an attempt to pull one of these plants free will only pull the plant in two, while the holdfast remains attached to the rock. Rocky shore plants often have gas-filled bladders which act to float the plant out into the current. Quite a few of these plants also have an extreme tolerance to drying, which is an adaptation to the shifting tide of a rocky shore. When exposed at low tide, these plants appear blackened and dead but regain a normal appearance when they are once again submerged.

Life Within and On Man

1. *Life within man.* A large number of organisms lead a parasitic life in our tissues and organs. In a way, this environment is less demanding than a rocky shore, for we offer a rather sheltered, tranquil

environment and an assured food supply. On the other hand, this environment has one very unsettling characteristic. Sooner or later it is bound to die, leaving its unfortunate inhabitants without a home. As a result, all human parasites have adapted themselves to this problem by developing ways of transferring their kind from one human host to another. Sometimes the process of transfer becomes very complex. The human pork tapeworm, *Taenia solium*, is a good example. The adult tapeworm lives in our small intestine. The worm's head, or *scolex*, is embedded in the intestinal wall and is held in place by four suckers. The worm has no digestive organs; it absorbs food directly into its body. The muscular and nervous systems are rudimentary and the body itself is divided into segments called *proglottids*. Each proglottid produces both sperm and eggs and is self-fertilizing. Proglottids are formed just behind the worm's head, so those near its tail are the oldest. Mature proglottids are filled almost solidly with developing eggs. A good-sized pork tapeworm may have up to two thousand proglottids and measure fifteen feet in length. When fully mature, proglottids break off and pass out with the host's feces. Almost all of the eggs thus shed will die, but a few will eventually be eaten by pigs. That this seemingly unlikely event will transpire is assured by the number of eggs produced; a typical proglottid contains eighty thousand

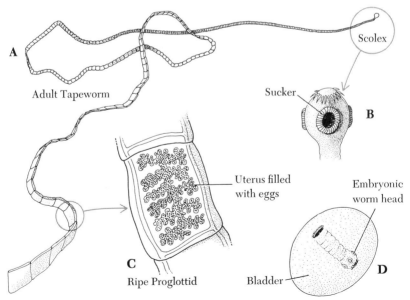

Figure 2-2. *Taenia solium,* the pork tapeworm. See text for details.

eggs, and an adult worm will shed eight to ten proglottids a day. Once inside a pig, the eggs form into small *bladders,* each containing an embryonic worm head. If we eat raw pork that is contaminated with these bladders, the heads will evert and attach to our intestine, completing the cycle.

Not all human parasites transfer their kind in as complex a fashion as does the pork tapeworm. Many bacteria and viruses are beautifully adapted to the conditions of our urban environment. Taking advantage of man's propensity to live in crowds, they transfer themselves from host to host in the droplets of a sneeze or cough.

2. *Life on man.* Those parasites which dwell on rather than within man have an additional problem—that of hanging on. Once again, adaptations have arisen to solve this problem. The human louse provides a good example. Three kinds of human lice are known. The *head louse* lives in the hair on man's head. The *crab louse* usually lives in man's pubic region, although sometimes it inhabits the eyebrows or the axillary hair of the armpit. The *body louse* lives in the fibers of man's clothing and is probably a latecomer to the group. Lice are adapted to maintain a tight grip on their uncertain environment. The louse's body is flattened and equipped with strong, grasping legs (Figure 2-3). Each leg has an ingeniously designed terminal claw which tightly grasps a hair or fiber. Interestingly, the legs of the pubic louse are adapted to grasp the larger hairs of the type occuring in that region. Lice lay their eggs on the lower portions of hairs or clothes fibers. The eggs, sometimes called *nits,* are cemented on and extremely difficult to remove.

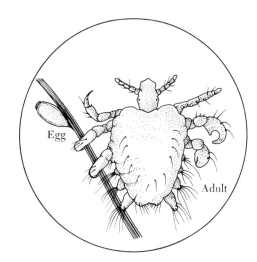

Figure 2-3. The human pubic louse. (After Faust, Ernest C., and P. F. Russell, *Clinical Parasitology.* Philadelphia: Lea and Febiger, 1965.)

A number of smaller organisms live directly on the human skin, but the skin is indeed a precarious environment. For one thing, dead cells are continually being shed. As Marples put it, "From the viewpoint of a microorganism on the skin (these) are enormous flat boulders of inert material, boulders that suddenly curl up and float away, bearing with them any organism that happens to be aboard." [5] At other times, the unfortunate microorganisms are subject to floods, scraping, and a host of other unpredictable hazards. The fauna and flora of our skin

THE IMPORTANCE OF A FRONT END

Since it is a sedentary, attached animal, hydra has no front end. This is true of attached animals in general and also of some mobile ones such as jellyfish or seastars. In animals of this kind, the nerve tissue is dispersed throughout the body. In contrast to hydras, jellyfish, or seastars, most animals do have a front end. This may seem a rather prosaic characteristic, but of all the developments within the stream of organic evolution, frontendedness is far and away the most significant. Some of the single-celled protozoa have a front end, but their microscopic size seems to have precluded development of organ systems and thus the potential that a front end presents. Among the larger multicellular animals, or metazoa, the story has been quite different. Even in very primitive metazoa such as the flatworm, sense receptors are concentrated in the front end or *head* as it might now be called. This concentration has obvious adaptive advantages, for it places the worm's receptors where they can best read the oncoming and largely unknown environment that the worm must continually explore. In a primitive metozoan such as the flatworm, the head has no brain. There is some nerve tissue associated with the sense receptors, but almost all of the nervous system is dispersed throughout the body, just as it is in the hydra.

Among higher metazoa, such as insects, the picture changes, for two highly significant developments have taken place. First, the sense organs of the head have become more complex and require more nerve tissue to process their input. Second, this nerve tissue has become fused into a true brain. Among the higher metazoa, this brain increasingly assumes the task of controlling all behavior. As a result, the nerve tissue scattered throughout the body assumes a secondary importance

are adapted to surmount these obstacles in various ways. Some, such as the follicle mites, survive by living in the tiny openings with which the skin is equipped. The bacteria which infest our skin overcome the problem by a high rate of reproduction, for even after the most thorough washing, our skin will soon be repopulated by the descendants of those few bacteria which have managed to survive.

Everywhere we look, we find evidence of adaptation in nature. To some, this is sure evidence of a supreme being, of an overriding purpose

in this respect. Once a true brain appears, the stage has been set for the next development, which is an evolutionary trend toward a brain that is progressively larger and more sophisticated until a critical threshold is reached—a brain capable of the insight and consciousness which characterizes the mind of man.

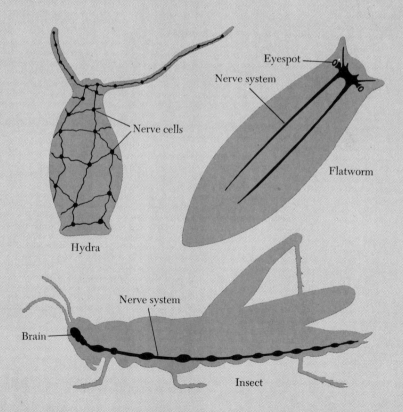

Eyespot

Nerve system

Nerve cells

Flatworm

Hydra

Nerve system

Brain

Insect

in the cosmos. To most biologists, it is better explained as a result of the process called natural selection.

NATURAL SELECTION

The theory of natural selection is built on three observations and one inference. The three observations are as follows:

1. *Life has a tremendous reproductive potential.* As energy-capturing machines, living things constantly seek to increase their own kind. One pair of houseflies can theoretically multiply to five trillion houseflies in five generations of unlimited breeding. Even elephants have a huge potential. As Charles Darwin calculated, a single pair of elephants could produce 19 million descendants in seven hundred fifty years. Man also has this potential, for one woman is theoretically capable of producing over sixty offspring.

2. *Plant and animal populations tend to remain constant.* Over short time periods, most plant and animal populations show fluctuations, often dramatic ones. Over longer periods, however, these fluctuations average out, and the population of most species remains fairly constant. Man seems to be an exception to this pattern, but it may well be that we are in for a rude surprise on this point.

3. *The individuals within a population vary.* No two organisms in a population are ever completely identical. If one were to collect hydras from a pond, some would have five tentacles, while others would have six or seven. Some (assuming one could relax them) would be longer than others. Tapeworms vary in the number of proglottids they produce; lice vary in their ability to effectively grasp human hairs. Variations such as these arise through mistakes or mutations in genes. Sometimes, variations are unique, producing a structure or behavior that has never appeared before.

It was Charles Darwin's great insight to realize that, taken together, these three observations implied that a process of *natural selection* must be taking place. Darwin reasoned that since plants and animals have a huge reproductive potential which is not realized, something must act to hold their numbers down. This something could only be a natural selection of those individuals best adapted to survive in their environments. All others would either be killed off or prevented from reproducing, thus holding plant and animal populations relatively constant from generation to generation.

Natural selection acts to weed out those individuals who have some weakness, who are less adapted to, or fit for, their environment than

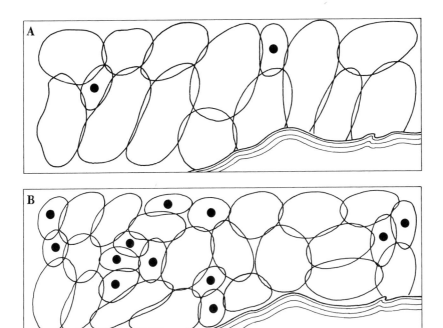

Figure 2-4. How territory size helps to hold reproduction down. A. The region shown has been divided into 15 territories. In all but two (with dots) male birds have attracted females. B. If 30 territories are crowded into the same region, almost half of the males, those with the smallest territories, will fail to attract mates.

are their luckier peers. Weakness can mean many things. Rocky shore animals release thousands of larval young, but only a very few survive. Some larvae are taken by predators. Others are dashed against rocks or swept out to sea. Still others fail to make a satisfactory attachment to the rocky shore. And those who do survive to adulthood are still subject to natural selection. If a barnacle settles in an isolated spot, it has been selected against as effectively as if it had never settled at all, for it is unable to contribute to the next generation. This is so because barnacles fertilize each other through a long penis. Thus, an isolated barnacle is effectively eliminated from reproduction. Sometimes a disease will take the more susceptible adults before they have had a chance to reproduce. In many situations, food is an effective agent of natural selection. If food is in short supply, those individuals who are weaker or in some way less adapted to their environment than others will be the first to starve.

Disease, food supply, and predators are all extrinsic agents of natural selection. Sometimes intrinsic agents operating within a population will also act as selective agents preventing the reproduction of weaker individuals and so holding the population's growth down. Many of these intrinsic means of natural selection are very subtle. If the flour beetles' environment becomes too crowded, beetles will begin to eat each other's eggs. In some species of frogs, chorusing at breeding time acts as an agent of natural selection. If too many frogs are present, the chorusing may be loud enough to prevent some females from reproducing, probably through an induced change in their reproductive systems. Many animals are territorial. Typically, males will claim and defend a territory. If too many males are present in one area, some will hold territories that are too small to attract females (Figure 2-4). Sometimes stress appears to act as a population-control mechanism. Rats kept under abnormally crowded conditions have been shown to develop odd behavior patterns which were apparently related to excessive stress and which prevented normal reproduction.

EVOLUTION

Over long periods of time, natural selection acts to create new species of plants and animals. We will give two examples of how this can take place.

1. *Industrial melanism.* By the 1850's, the Midlands of England had become transformed. Once an agricultural region, the Midlands became the heart of England's burgeoning industrial revolution. Cities such as Manchester spewed out pollution, and the countryside became covered with coal smoke from hundreds of factories.

There are over seven hundred different species of moths in England, many of which can be found in the Midlands. Some of these are active at night and rest on tree trunks during the day. Over one hundred years ago biologists began to notice that many of the nocturnal species in the Midlands area seemed to be changing from their former light gray color to a darker *melanistic* shade. Extensive investigation has shown this to be a result of natural selection acting within a changing environment. As pollution in the Midlands increased, tree trunks became blackened with coal smoke and soot. Under earlier conditions a pale color was highly adaptive, for moths were well concealed on trees where they would blend into the light-colored lichens which encrusted the tree trunks. But when the pollution blackened tree trunks and killed the lichens, the light-colored moths were no longer concealed and fell easy prey to various predators. Occasional melanistic variants with a darker coloration had always been present in moth populations but had been at a selective disadvantage. With the advent

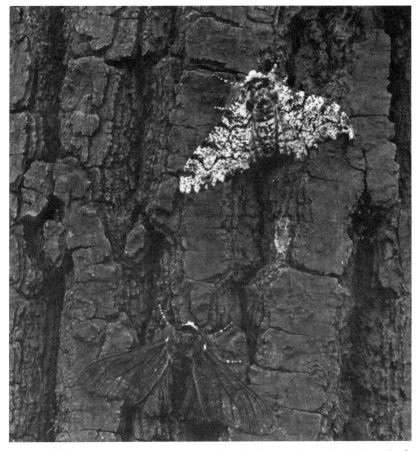

Figure 2-5. The peppered moth *Biston betularia* and its melanic form both seen on a soot-covered oak trunk near Birmingham, England. (From the experiments of Dr. H.B.D. Kettlewell, University of Oxford.)

of pollution, this particular variant was now at an advantage, and a strong natural selection for melanism took place. It has been possible to document this change with great accuracy. In 1850, for example, almost all individuals of one species, the peppered moth, were pale in color. Now the peppered moths about Manchester are almost uniformly melanistic. The Manchester environment has probably had other effects on the local peppered moth population, for there is evidence that melanistic moths differ from pale ones in certain behavioral and physiological traits. Should the Manchester population become isolated from pale populations of peppered moth and should this isolation continue for a long enough time, a phenomenon called *reproductive isolation* could occur. When this happens, two populations within a single species have become so different that they will not cross to produce offspring even if the barrier which separates them is removed. The result is then a new species of moth.

2. *Venereal syphilis.* The *Treponema* bacteria is responsible for a number of diseases. Pinta is a skin infection common throughout the tropics. Yaws, also common in the tropics, is an ulcerative skin disease which can affect the bones. Endemic syphilis, or bejel, is another tropical skin disease which also affects the bones. All three of these treponeme diseases are caused by casual contact. The fourth treponeme disease, venereal syphilis, differs from the others in that it is transmitted almost exclusively by sexual intercourse. C.J. Hackett and other scientists have made a strong case for the evolution of all four variants from a common ancestor. Hackett believes pinta arose first, then yaws and then endemic syphilis. He thinks the last variant, venereal syphilis, emerged in the developing cities of Asia and the Near East around five thousand years ago. As Europe became urbanized, venereal syphilis

THE TERMITE COLONY AS A SUPERORGANISM

A new termite colony is started by a *royal pair* of termites who leave an established colony. After excavating a nest, the pair does nothing but reproduce. Stored fat, plus protein from their now useless flight muscles, nourish the royal pair until their young are able to gather food. Large numbers of eggs are produced; the queens of some tropical species can lay up to twenty thousand eggs a day. The eggs develop into immature termites called *nymphs*. Each nymph has the potential of developing into a soldier, a worker, or a supplementary reproductive. Soldiers defend the colony. They have enormous jaws and, in some species, a head shaped to fit tightly into colony entranceways, thus blocking out invaders. Workers build nests, collect food, and tend the eggs. A third sort of adult, the supplementary reproductive, will produce young after the royal pair dies.

The number of each kind or caste of adult is tightly regulated by the colony. This can be shown experimentally. If, for example, a large number of soldiers is removed, a higher percentage of nymphs will become soldiers until the imbalance is corrected. If the royal pair is removed from a colony, supplementary reproductives will arise to take their place. Most colonies tolerate only one reproductive pair at a time. If a reproductive pair is removed and then reintroduced to the colony after a new pair has been formed, the excess pair will be killed.

spread northward, taking advantage of the routes opened by trade and warfare. Venereal syphilis has one great advantage over the other treponeme diseases. Since the treponemes are sensitive to cold, those strains which cause pinta, yaws, and endemic syphilis are largely limited to the tropics or to moderate climates. Because it is spread by sexual intercourse, the venereal variant does not face this limitation. It is thus a new strain of *Treponema* which has been able to exploit colder environments which remain closed to the other strains. The result is an effective isolation between treponeme populations, which probably will lead to a species difference between the organisms causing yaws, pinta, and endemic syphilis and the organism responsible for venereal syphilis (Figure 2-6).

Over millions of years, the process of natural selection has given rise to literally millions of species. Figure 2-7A shows an evolutionary tree for the animal kingdom, one way of depicting the specia-

As you have no doubt noticed, there are some striking similarities between a termite colony and a hydra.

1. Both are started by a royal pair. In hydra, the royal pair are *gametes*, a single egg and spermatozoon.

2. The units which make up a termite colony or a hydra are initially undifferentiated or unspecialized. In one case these are young cells; in the other, nymphs.

3. Both a hydra and a termite colony maintain a close regulation over the kind and the number of specialized units they contain. In other words, both are homeostatic integrated systems, in which the units, whether cells or termites, are subordinate to the interests of the system as a whole. In a hydra, this regulation is maintained by chemicals which move between cells. A termite colony also employs chemicals to regulate its members. These chemicals are *social hormones* sometimes called *pheromones*. Termites pass these chemicals to each other by their antennae so that, in effect, they act as a chemical language.

4. Both hydra and a termite colony are energy-capturing systems designed to take matter and energy from their surroundings in order to build more of their own kind.

5. Both are automatic systems under genetic control.

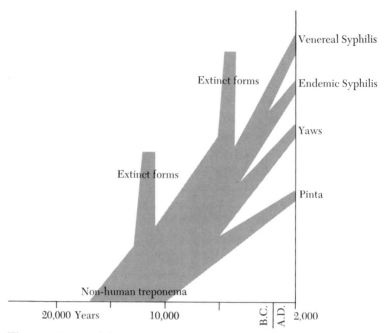

Figure 2-6. A syphilis "family tree," showing hypothetical relationships between different forms of the treponeme diseases. (After Brothwell, Don, "The Real History of Syphilis," *Science Journal,* 6, September 1970, pp. 27–32.)

tion which has taken place since life first arose. As the figure indicates, biologists divide the evolutionary tree into major branches or *phyla.* These represent groups of plants or animals which have basic similarities in structure and are thus presumed to be more closely related to each other than to the species in other phyla.

On first examination, evolution might seem to be a completely random process; however, this is not so, for at least two trends can be identified.

1. *Expansion.* As the tree suggests, life has expanded through time. This expansion has covered the earth with a thin film of life sometimes called the *biosphere.* The expansion can be measured either in terms of *biomass,* that is, total bulk of life, or it can be measured in terms of species numbers. In the latter case, the expansion rate has varied from phylum to phylum. Interestingly, the chordate phylum, to which we belong, has been on the decline for some time (Figure 2-7B).

2. *Complexity.* As one moves up along the evolutionary tree, organisms tend to have an increasingly complex structure and be-

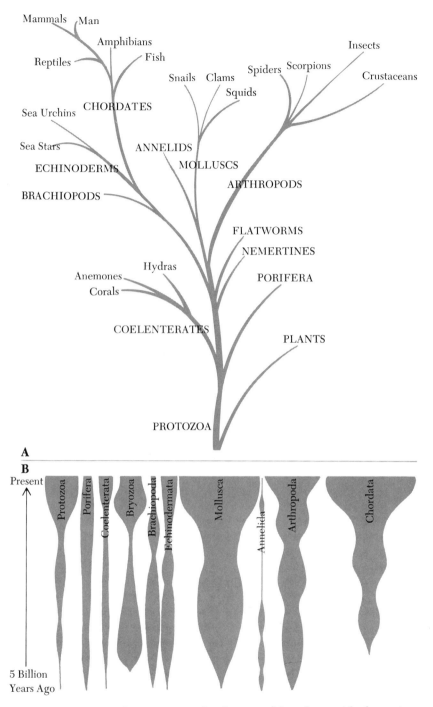

Figure 2-7. A. An evolutionary tree for the animal kingdom, with the major phyla in capital letters. B. Each of the major phyla in terms of its variety of forms through time. Note that the Chordata, to which man belongs, have shown some recent decline.

31

havior. Because of this, they generally are more vulnerable to disruption. The behavior of higher organisms is more sophisticated and is directed by an increasingly centralized nerve system. In higher organisms a larger percentage of behavior is learned and less is genetic or instinctive. Lower organisms typically produce many young, few of which survive to adulthood. Higher organisms, in contrast, tend to produce fewer offspring with a higher survival rate.

Taken together, these trends suggest that life is *opportunistic*. In its drive to capture energy and matter from the environment and convert these into organized living tissues, life has expanded into all available environments and has taken advantage of new opportunities presented to it. The evolutionary record also suggests that this opportunistic expansion has been successful largely because life has continually increased in sophistication and complexity.

Does the opportunism of evolution imply that it has a purpose? Recall that living things have the characteristic of homeostasis. That is, when disturbed, they show a goal-seeking or purposeful behavior, for they return to their normative form. Since evolution is a product of living things, one might expect that it, too, would exhibit some sort of purposeful or goal-seeking behavior. To the biologist Conrad Waddington, evolution does indeed have this characteristic. Waddington uses the term *chreod*, which is derived from the Greek words meaning *necessary path*, when he talks about the goal-seeking behavior of evolution. An automatic pilot is a chreodic system, guiding a plane along a preset flight path, and so is a computer-run assembly line. In the realm of life, an embryo is a chreodic system, for the adult form is programmed within the embryo's genes. Is evolution a chreodic system, destined also to move toward some end point? To some, the end point of evolution is man. To others, man is only another one of evolution's products, some day to be superceded by other, perhaps more sophisticated forms of life. Regardless of his particular view of evolution, almost every student of man agrees that at this point in time man is dominant on earth, largely because of culture, his new adaptive dimension. Who were man's immediate ancestors, and what selective pressures led to the advent of man himself and his unique power to build cultures? We consider these questions in the next two chapters.

3 MAN'S PRIMATE ANCESTORS

Obviously, we have no way of observing our ancestors directly. The best we can do is to rely on evidence from fossil material and from the study of our primate relatives, the great apes. From these sources anthropologists have built the following very tentative yet generally agreed upon picture of man's ancestors: They lived in tropical or subtropical regions of Africa and perhaps Asia. In general appearance they resembled a modern great ape such as the chimpanzee. Hairy, tailless, semierect in posture, they were somewhat smaller than modern man. Although they had a potential life span of around thirty years, this was rarely reached, for the selective agents of predation, famine, accident, and disease took a heavy toll. Our ancestors were accomplished tree climbers and spent much, perhaps most, of their lives in the trees of their forest environment. As with all tree-dwelling members of the primate group, they had a well developed grasping hand and stereoscopic vision, adaptations which enabled them to move from branch to branch and tree to tree. The exceptional skill necessary for survival in the trees had given rise to a brain able to coordinate eye and hand movement. Their higher brain or cerebral cortex was particularly well developed.

Our apelike ancestors probably spent some time on the ground, and although awkward at it, they could walk for limited distances. This inference is supported by observations of wild chimpanzees and other contemporary primates. Jane van Lawick-Goodall, for example, reports seeing chimpanzees gathering wild fruits into their arms and then walking short distances to a desired spot before eating them.

Our ancestors probably ranged over their habitat in bands of ten to thirty. Each band occupied a roughly defined territory which centered on a home nest or nests. The bands were scattered throughout the forests and probably contacted each other only at infrequent intervals. Each band would typically consist of one or a few males, several females, and a number of young. Males would be sexually interested in any receptive female and mating would not be restricted to periods when females were in *estrus* or heat. Births normally were single and the young would be nursed, protected, and reared by the mother, with the male parent taking relatively little interest in them other than in a general sense as protector of the band. Those young who were malformed or diseased would be left by the band to die. Band members tended to move together for security. Intraband conflict was probably infrequent, with the largest male having dominance

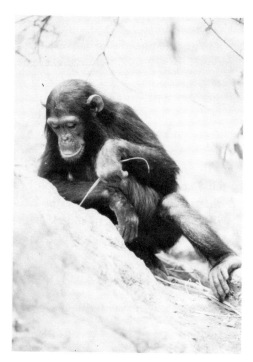

Figure 3-1. A five-year-old chimpanzee in Tanzania's Gombe Stream Reserve uses a blade of grass to fish for termites. (Photo by Baron Hugo van Lawick; © National Geographic Society.)

over the others. A kind of pecking order or dominance sequence probably existed so that most individuals knew their relative status within the band. Mutual band activity such as the grooming and play seen among chimpanzees probably helped to hold the group together. Communication was by physical pushing and prodding or by vocal calls and signals.

Were these ancestors of ours tool users? This is a question of critical importance, since the ability to use tools is closely associated with the rise of man.

Although the use of tools is rather rare among modern primates other than man, it does occur. Chimpanzees will use a stick to extract termites from their nests. At certain times of the year, the normally thick walls of African termite nests are thinned down by the termites, who drill holes to prepare for their emergence at mating time. Chimpanzees will take advantage of this by inserting sticks into the holes and then licking off the termites which collect on the sticks. Apparently chimpanzees plan ahead or use foresight in their termite collecting, for they have been observed to carry a stick for a mile or more while looking for suitable termite nests. Presumably our primate ancestors also used tools of this sort, including stones, which would be used as weapons or crude hammers.

Although their well-developed brains and ability to use tools made our primate ancestors among the most sophisticated of the forest dwellers, the species was still just another member of the forest ecosystem, bound into its cycle along with hundreds of other species. Our ancestors were largely primary consumers, that is, vegetarians. Perhaps eighty per cent of their food consisted of plant material. Their dental pattern resembled that found in modern apes, and they had large canines which served to tear the tough rinds of fruits. Some animal food was taken, which probably consisted of small, slow game and grubs, snails, or similar creatures which might be found as the band moved through the forest.

In summary, then, our ancestors probably had the following key characteristics. They possessed a well-developed brain which was coupled with exceptional coordination of hand and eye. They followed a nomadic band life in the trees, with occasional forays onto the ground. Their diet was omnivorous, and food gathering probably involved some tool use and even a rudimentary kind of foresight. All of these characteristics were traits which were destined to be of vital importance in the evolutionary step to man.

A large number of books and articles deal with the evidence for this tentative picture of man's ancestors. A sampling of these is listed in the bibliography.

4

THE EVOLUTION OF MAN

Man's ancestors had evolved a successful life style. Life in the trees was relatively stable and secure. What happened, then, to change all this and start those selective pressures which ultimately led to the evolution of man? This has always been one of the most difficult questions for anthropologists to answer. What follows is a majority view as to the probable sequence of events which led to man.

Over two million years ago, extended periods of drought probably began to reduce those forests which sheltered man's ancestors. In the course of hundreds of thousands of years a similar pattern must have occurred over and over. Forests would become thinned into groves of trees which could no longer support all of the bands in the region. Some of the weaker ones would be forced out into the surrounding open country, or savannah, to perish, or, if they were lucky, to make their way to another grove and regain the safety of the trees. The savannah must have been a forbidding place—full of large, swift, hostile animals and lacking in shelter, water, or familar foods. Our immediate ancestors were thus evolutionary failures; they were the ones who could not compete effectively enough to keep a foothold in the trees. Most of the dispossessed probably perished, but some survived, and a few of these dispossessed bands came to spend increasing periods on the savannah. Among them, a complex of powerful selective forces was at work. Natural selection caused certain characteristics to become more and more common among our ancestral ground-dwelling bands. Many of these characteristics had been present in rudimentary form among man's tree-dwelling ancestors. Although we can only speculate, it seems likely that the adaptations to savannah life which we will now describe developed as a complex pattern rather than as a simple sequence.

Adaptation to a savannah existence produced a series of physical changes. Among these were loss of body hair, most probably as a result of the increased activity associated with savannah life; a dark pigment to ward off excessive sun; and certain facial changes, in particular the reduction of jaw size. A dramatic increase in brain size took place. Until recently, many anthropologists thought that this brain enlargement led to the appearance of human traits. Now it seems more likely that an increase in brain size followed or at most accompanied the other adaptive changes associated with savannah life. The reason for this view is the realization that something must have forced the brain to enlarge, for a large brain carries certain disadvantages. It requires much blood (twelve per cent of the total body's blood in modern man), all of which must be pumped uphill. It also enlarges the head, leading to problems at birth.

Once on the ground, those of our ancestors who could see and run from danger before it was too late obviously would be favored for survival. Such an individual would have good eyesight; he would be active and perceptive and stand erect. The latter characteristic would not only allow its bearer to rise above the savannah grass to survey his surroundings; it would also lead to the development of carrying ability, an adaptation which would prove to be of crucial importance in coping with savannah life. When still in the trees, man's ancestors certainly used their hands to carry and manipulate objects, but the continual need to grasp branches while moving from tree to tree made this at best a secondary and occasional function of the hands. For a ground-dwelling bipedal animal the situation now would be completely different. The hands would be free for all kinds of new functions, the most important being the ability to carry objects. In moving from spot to spot, food, infants, tools, and other objects could now be carried. At first, band members scavenging an animal carcass or collecting plants might simply eat their fill and move on. Later, particularly if surprised by a potential predator, they might grab a portion and run. One can imagine a transition from a grab-and-run behavior to one in which scavenged meat or gathered plants were removed and carried back to a home camp for use by the band. Those

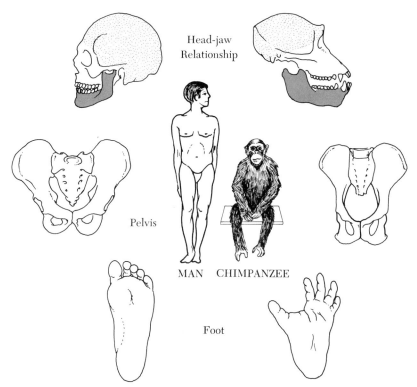

Figure 4-1. Some adaptations associated with upright posture. Brain-case enlarges relative to jaw, pelvis broadens to support overlying viscera, and foot changes from grasping to supportive organ.

bands which developed this behavior would certainly have an adaptive advantage.

In addition to the use of hands to carry things, life on the savannah created selective pressures which led to another adaptive novelty— the ability to hand-fashion tools. A carcass can be much more effectively dismembered with a sharpened rock than with one's teeth, and roots are more easily extracted with a digging stick than by hand. Although our tree-dwelling ancestors probably had some ability to use tools, this had been an intermittent and casual behavior. Now tool use could often be the difference between survival and death. One can imagine many such situations. The surprised forager who grabs a rock and stuns an attacking animal will live to pass his genes along, while his less capable companion will not. The mother who can fill gourds with water and carry them back to her family will have water to see

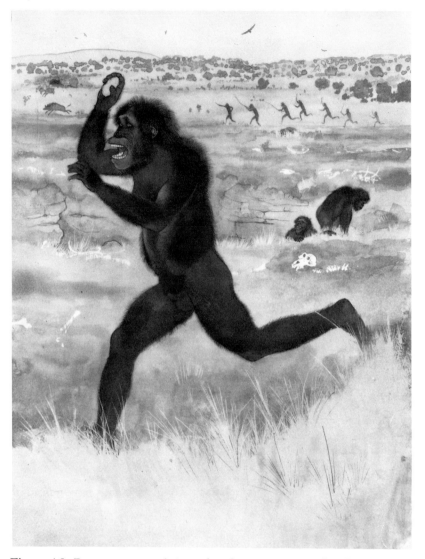

Figure 4-2. Reconstruction of *Australopithecus,* a genus related to man, or
Homo sapiens. Australopithecus ranged African savannas from one half
to five million years ago. Considerable evidence exists to suggest he was
a tool user. (Courtesy of the Trustees of the British Museum of Natural
History.)

them through days of drought, while her sister who is less endowed
with the knack of fashioning things will perish along with her children.

Another trait inevitably accompanies carrying and tool use—the
capacity to look ahead, to plan. Man's tree-dwelling ancestors prob-

ably had some limited foresight. On the savannah this trait became of crucial importance, for only a creature with foresight will carry food back to a camp or carry a digging stick in anticipation of coming across a succulent root.

Successful life on the savannah led to still another set of fundamental changes. It became necessary for our ancestors, rather than subsisting on a plant diet, to rely to a much larger extent on animal foods. The behavior patterns which accompanied a successful adaptation to the new savannah foods were of profound importance. Bands would now utilize a greater diversity of food material, ranging from plants and small animals to larger hunted species. This meant the development of a wide range of hunting-gathering techniques. As a result, these early savannah dwellers were much more versatile than their ancestors and more versatile than most other animals. As one anthropologist has noted, only two mammalian species—man and the brown rat—have managed to colonize the world, and both are omnivorous.

Selective pressures for a successful life on the savannah also led to basic changes in the social life of the band. Sexual promiscuity, the most probable pattern among our tree-dwelling ancestors, was now replaced by pair bonding, a social pattern in which one male establishes a settled sexual relationship with one female. This kind of relationship led to greater efficiency and security. The males did most of the hunting, while a large portion of the women's time was devoted to gathering and child care. The increasing complexity of band life necessitated a much longer training period for infants than was true for life in the trees.

Hunting large game, child-rearing, tool-making, all required an increased ability to cooperate, to get along as a group. Of all the new savannah adaptations, the ability to cooperate was perhaps the most crucial, and this trait must have been strongly selected for.

Cooperation, however, can only be carried so far if one must communicate solely by grunts, pushes, and gestures. The pressure for more efficient communication which flowed from the new needs of a savannah band was accompanied by a fortunate happenstance. With the use of hands to carry things, the mouth would be free—to chatter. Sooner or later this chatter and its signals for danger or opportunity evolved into a language, an ability to express ideas in symbolic form. Language had tremendous adaptive value for savannah life, and one could argue that its appearance was the single most crucial event of all the changes taking place in savannah dwellers. The appearance and spread of speech had a profound effect on band social life. It was now possible to transmit information in the form of tradition, and the elders within a band might well take on increased stature as the keepers of this tradition. It was also possible to pass along information about tool-making, hunting techniques, and a myriad of other items from generation to generation. In short, our savannah dwellers would now be carriers of a culture.

To sum up: Bipedalism, carrying, tool use, a wide-ranging diet, foresight, cooperation, and symbolic communication were all adaptations for a hunting-gathering savannah existence. Their survival value led to a strong selection for individuals genetically endowed with these traits and produced a new sort of creature, different in kind from all other living things. Although emergent man still retained most of the basic characteristics of his ancestors, his ability to create a culture was an evolutionary breakthrough and marked the beginning of a new way of living, unlike any seen before.

5 CULTURE

How can culture best be defined? The great English anthropologist, Edward Burnett Tylor, defined culture as "that complex whole which includes knowledge, belief, art, morals, law, custom, and any other capabilities and habits acquired by man as a member of society." [6] A more recent definition by the anthropologist Ashley Montagu is: "With the creation and usage of organized systems of symbols man created a new dimension of experience . . . we call *culture*. Culture is man-made. It is the environment which man creates in order the better to control as much of the environment as he desires." [7]

These definitions share the idea that culture is a man-made, learned activity. In order to appreciate fully the importance of this learning, imagine what would happen if a member of some primitive culture, such as a Kalahari Bushman, were catapulted into a typical American town, arriving in the business district on a Saturday afternoon. Obviously, he might cause some upset among pedestrians, but their upset would be nothing compared to his. Anthropologists have told of their rather eerie sensation of unease upon confronting a completely alien culture for the first time; our Bushman would be more than uneasy— he would probably be terrified. Of course, he would see and feel some familiar things. He would recognize the sun, recognize the water in a drinking fountain, perhaps experience a familiar sympathy for a crying child. On the other hand, the larger part of this new environment would be unfamiliar. Its unfamiliar aspects would consist largely of objects, activities, and ideas which collectively we could label *Western culture*. The Bushman would have no way of understanding these objects, ideas, and activities. He might make some inferences, using traits of his own culture as a base, but his culture is so different from ours that it would offer little help. Certainly nothing coded in the Bushman's genes could help him. The Bushman would be overwhelmed by an unending series of objects and happenings, all without any meaning to him. How would he react to a green traffic light, a policeman's whistle, a sign reading "Keep Off the Grass"? The continuous jabbering of passing pedestrians would offer him no clues as to what could or could not be done, what was considered friendly or hostile behavior, what the gestures of an approaching man meant, or what purposes were served by the innumerable objects he encountered around him.

Sooner or later our struggling Bushman would come under the wing of some person or group, and a process of organized learning would begin. This would largely entail mastering the *symbolic* meaning of objects and acts. A car, for example, is simply a tangle of materials until we learn of its meaning as an object of transport, prestige, and excitement. The word *great* is a meaningless sound until we have learned to associate it with certain emotions. In a similar way the Bushman would come to learn the symbolic meanings of a green traffic light, a policeman's whistle, and a thousand other cultural elements.

Our culture is thus not only learned, it is also symbolic. Some recent work suggests that chimpanzees can be taught to use symbols. Yet their ability to attach symbolic meanings to things remains far below that of man.

In addition to being learned and symbolic, culture has another property of great importance which has to do with the way it is learned. Animals often teach one another, but our teaching is of an entirely different order. For one thing, we increasingly teach on an impersonal basis, using media such as the newspapers or TV. This means that the ideas of a culture can be spread very rapidly, much more rapidly than the learned information which animals transmit to each other.

Culture also tends to be cumulative. Ideas and capabilities developed hundreds of years ago, and perhaps no longer believed in or practiced, can be and often are carried down from generation to generation.

The concept of evolution can be applied not only to the biological, but also to the cultural realm, for it is possible to build an evolutionary tree for cultures as well as for organisms. Biological and cultural evolution resemble each other in two important ways. First, both fight the entropy which characterizes the universe. Second, both systems have tended to grow. In biological evolution, this growth has been one of increase in the total bulk, kinds, and complexity of organisms. In cultural evolution it has been a growth of ideas and material objects.

Biological and cultural evolution differ in two important ways. First, the innovations of biological evolution are transmitted through genetic inheritance, while those of cultural evolution are transmitted through symbols. Second, since symbols are a much faster and more efficient way of transmitting information than are genes, the ideas and the material objects which form the stream of cultural evolution have accumulated and changed much more rapidly than have the organisms of biological evolution (Figure 5-1).

Unlike any other organism, man is the product of two evolutionary systems, his innate biological one and his learned cultural one. It is

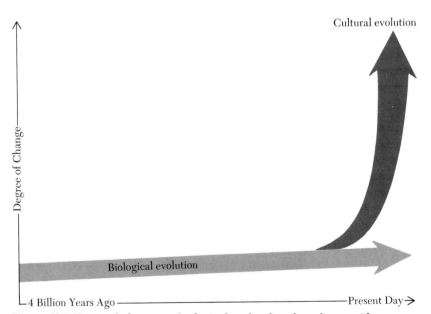

Figure 5-1. Rates of change in biological and cultural evolution. Change in biological evolution has been very slow and has proceded at a more or less even rate. In contrast, cultural change has been rapid, and has accelerated through time.

important, however, to realize that in everyday life man's biological and his cultural characteristics are tightly intertwined and it is often difficult to tell whether a given trait is biological or cultural in origin. Sometimes this can be done with reasonable success. For example, most white adults, about ninety-five per cent, can drink cow's milk without trouble. In contrast, most nonwhites suffer intestinal upset shortly after they take any sizeable amount of milk. Since milk is a staple food for many white adults but not for other races, it might seem that this difference is a learned one. Further investigation, however, has revealed that whites have an enzyme, lactase, which digests the lactose sugar present in cow's milk. Nonwhite adults lack this enzyme so that the lactose sugar goes unchanged to the large intestine, where it is attacked by bacteria, producing intestinal upset. This would seem to suggest that an innate biological difference, rather than a cultural one, is involved. Presumably, a natural selection for the presence of the lactase enzyme has been coupled with thousands of years of milk drinking among white peoples.

More often than not, however, man's traits are a result of both cul-

IS HUMAN SOCIETY A SUPERORGANISM?

An earlier box compared a termite colony with hydra. Both were found to be homeostatic, integrated, reproducing, energy-capturing systems.

The great English sociologist Herbert Spencer thought of human society as an organism too—a *superorganism.* In his work *Principles of Sociology,* Spencer listed these similarities between an organism and human society.

1. Both grow.
2. As they increase in size, both increase in complexity. An embryo has few parts, as does a young society. Just as do adult organisms, mature societies have many parts. We call these parts classes, roles, or institutions.
3. Both organism and society show division of labor. They also show an integration and interdependence of units. In one case the units are cells; in the other, people.
4. In both, the whole outlives its units. Cells or individuals die, but organisms and societies live on.

tural and biological influences. This is particularly true in the case of complex characteristics; intelligence is a well known example.

Culture consists of ideas and beliefs, of material objects, and of the know-how to obtain the latter. The term *technology* is commonly used for all those methods a culture employs to take things from nature and turn them into useful material objects. Some animals have a kind of technology, for they are able to build things such as nests or sand-grain shells. Animal technology is largely instinctive and its products do not accumulate but cycle back into nature upon the death of their users. In contrast, man's technology is learned. It is also cumulative; that is, it has the capacity to increase steadily in its bulk, its complexity, and in its ability to wrest materials from nature. For over ninety per cent of his existence on earth, man has lived with a hunting-gathering technology. Only in the last fraction of his history has a new machine technology appeared, a technology which has drastically changed man's way of life. Before we look at this machine technology, we will take a detailed look at the Bushmen, who are one of very few hunting-gathering cultures still remaining on earth.

Are there any important differences between society and an organism?

To Spencer there was one critical difference. In the organism, consciousness is concentrated in one small region, the brain. In contrast, all the units, that is the people, of a society have, as he put it, "the capacities for happiness and misery."

The cells of a hydra and the termites of a termite colony are nameless and have no individuality, no fears or dreams. They are completely subordinate to the interests of the system to which they belong. Man is obviously different; our societies are supposedly built to serve the individuals they contain. Some biologists see this as part of an evolutionary trend from a nameless autonomy toward a greater and greater individualism. If so, this trend raises a crucial question: Is it possible to reconcile our individualism which we value so highly with the fact that to date all successful life systems have shown a high degree of homeostasis and integration, a subordination of unit to whole? We will return to this fundamental issue in Part III of the book.

6 THE BUSHMEN: A CULTURE WITH A HUNTING−GATHERING TECHNOLOGY

Most of the fifty-five thousand South African Bushmen who survive today live in settled communities. However, a few nomadic bands still exist in the Kalahari Desert (Figure 6-1). Archaeological records show that Bushmen once were scattered across South Africa, and the Kalahari bands are isolated remnants of a way of life once followed by all mankind.

The bands occupy a forbidding region. For nine months of the year, from March to December, the Kalahari is a desert. During the hot months of this period the wind dies out, the last of the surface water dries up, and the temperature may rise to 120°F. or more. In the cold months, June and July, water left in containers can freeze at night, and bitter winds sweep up from the Antarctic. December marks the beginning of the wet season; torrential rains bring a brief bloom of desert plants. By March, however, the rains have ceased and the ground begins to dry so that by June only a few scattered water holes remain, and these soon dry up.

In spite of its inhospitable nature, a variety of plants and animals have become adapted to life in the Kalahari. Wetter areas have tall grass and scattered trees. Even in the driest regions a few plants are found. These, particularly melons and root plants of various kinds, form the bulk of the Bushmen's diet. The Kalahari also has antelope, giraffe, ostrich, zebra, and the great cats which prey upon them, as well as

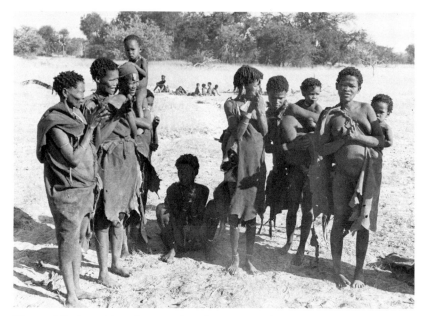

Figure 6-1. A social gathering of Bushwomen and children. Note open, semi-arid landscape. (Courtesy of the South African Information Service.)

the hyena, the jackal, and other large animals. A variety of smaller animals such as snakes, lizards, locusts, and bees have become adapted to the harsh demands of life in this region.

The Bushman band is actually an extended family. A typical band consists of about twenty people—perhaps an elderly couple, their daughters, and their daughters' husbands and children. Except on rare occasions when several bands come together, the typical Bushman lives in association with a relatively small group. As a consequence, a Bushman's relationship with his fellow man is almost always on a personal level. From continual daily contact he comes to know the strengths and weaknesses, the personality quirks of his fellow band members, just as we know those of our own families.

BELIEFS

The Bushman's relationship with the environment about him is also a personal one. Bushmen live in an animistic, supernatural world. It is *animistic* because they believe that the whole world of nature— animals, rocks, stars—behaves as men do, with their desires, emotions, fears, and multifarious purposes. It is *supernatural* because innumerable spirits and strange beings people this world. Here, for example, is the way one Kalahari band, the Kung Bushmen, describes the movement of the sun.

At night when the sun sets, the people with no knees catch it and kill it, for the sun is meat. They put it in a pot, and when it is cooked they tell their children to run off and play, and when the children are gone the people with no knees eat it. When the children come back, the people with no knees pick their teeth and give what they remove to the children, and then the people with no knees take the shoulder blade of the sun and throw it back into the east again, where a new sun grows and rises in the morning. If a tall man throws it you are aware of nothing, but if a short man throws it you can hear it whirring overhead.[8]

The Kung see themselves as a part of this animistic and supernatural world, intimately connected to all of its inhabitants by a network of mutual influence. A Kung believes that at birth he acquires a sort of essence, his *now*, which will forever connect him with nature in many different ways. For example, some people have wet nows, and when one of these people urinates into a fire, rain will come. But if someone with a dry now urinates into a fire, the rain will stop.

Bushmen also place death within a web of supernatural belief. The moon, for example, is hollow in its first quarter because it is carrying spirits of the dead; the hair of a dead person becomes a cloud; his bile colors the sky green.

The Bushman's belief system is essentially static. Although on occasion new spirits may come to be recognized or old ones fade from memory, the general patterns of belief are passed unchanged from generation to generation.

Bushmen have no sense of time as Westerners understand the word. Aside from a general awareness of seasons and other natural cycles, time is a meaningless concept—there are no clocks to watch, no schedules to meet. Time is not a scare commodity, to be gained or saved. Unlike the typical Westerner, the Bushman does not see growth, progress, or the accumulation of material goods as meaningful goals. As his culture is neither time- nor change-oriented, there is no sense of a distant past or of a promised land which lies ahead.

TECHNOLOGY

What is a hunting-gathering technology like and how does it wrest materials from nature? Since food-getting is the one most important

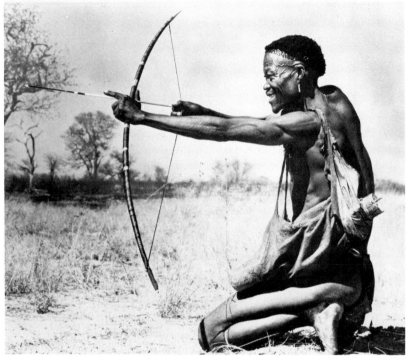

Figure 6-2. A Bushman hunter. (Courtesy of the South African Information Service.)

function of any technology, we will look in some detail at how the Bushmen obtain their food.

Among the Bushmen, hunting is normally the job of the men, and gathering, that of the women and children.

Although some groups use throwing sticks or spears, the bow and arrow is most commonly used in hunting. The bows are small and made of roughly shaped wood, the string either of sinew or wood fiber. Arrows are of wood, arrowheads of bone or iron. The Bushman's bow and arrow is a fragile weapon and rarely would kill were it not for the poisons the hunter applies to the tip and shaft of the arrow. These poisons are made of a wide variety of substances, such as vegetable juices, snake venom, or mashed beetle grubs. None of these poisons have an instantaneous effect, and Bushmen must pursue a wounded animal until it collapses. Although the Bushmen are a small people of rather thin build, they are capable of surprising strength and endurance and will often track wounded game for hours and sometimes for a day or more without pause.

Each Bushman knows his territory intimately—every bush, every melon patch, every hiding place for game. When tracking game, a hunter can tell what the animal is doing, whether it is running or making for water or feeding in a leisurely manner. A Bushman hunter is very careful in his dealings with nature. For example, he will follow a successful kill with a scarification ritual, in which he causes scars to form on his body by rubbing burnt flesh from the animal he has killed into wounds he makes on his arms or chest. This, he believes, will transfer some of the animal's strength to him and make him a better hunter. On the other hand, he will never take honey touched by a baboon because he believes that it will kill him.

When a kill is made, nothing is wasted. In her account of Bushman life, Elizabeth Thomas describes the preparation of a female gemsbok, a species of small antelope. First the Bushmen stripped her udder and drank the milk. Then the antelope's skin was cut free and placed in a shallow pit which served to catch all juices from the carcass. The antelope was cut up and all its parts distributed. Both the animal's blood and the liquid from its stomach were drunk. At the end of the butchering all that remained unused was a small pile of grass and other food from the stomach and intestines of the gemsbok.

A digging stick is the only tool a woman uses when she is out in the desert collecting plants. A variety of foods is sought out and placed into folds of the woman's cloak, or *kaross*. Among the foods collected are melons which grow in clusters on the ground, nuts, and succulent roots from many plant species. As do their men, the women have an intimate knowledge of their territory; they know where each melon patch and even each root-bearing vine grows. Elizabeth Thomas describes this closeness to nature which seems so phenomenal to Western eyes:

> We wandered about haphazardly for a time, looking for a vine, and presently I saw one twisted around some grass blades, binding them together in a tuft. I pointed it out to her, but she smiled and shook her head, turning her hands palm upwards in the gesture for nothing. She meant that it was a useless species of vine, marking nothing below. Later, as we walked along, she laughed. Twikwe was charmed by the mistakes the members of our expedition made, for they were always elementary and, to her, very diverting.[9]

Everything is used, nothing wasted. Tsama melons, for example, provide much more than just food. Their rinds can be made into bowls, cooking utensils, children's toys, or even resonators for musical instruments. Above all, the tsama's pulp yields water, a resource of vital importance in the dry season.

Sometimes a band will specialize in one kind of food source. Some northwest Kalahari Bushman bands which have recently been studied provide a good example of this.

These bands would always locate their camps near a water supply. In the season of rains, temporary pools were everywhere and the bands were scattered. In the dry season these temporary ponds dried up and water was restricted to eight permanent water holes. The bands responded by coming together at these locations.

The larger part of their food, over sixty per cent, was made up of vegetables. While some eighty-four species of edible plants are found in the region, one food, the nut from mongongo trees, formed from one-half to two-thirds of their vegetable diet. A typical Bushman would eat about three hundred of these nuts a day, the caloric equivalent of two and one-half pounds of cooked rice and the protein equivalent of fourteen ounces of lean beef. Whenever possible, camps were located within a short distance of a mongongo forest. Gathering of mongongo nuts and other vegetables was largely women's work and required little by way of equipment—some stones to crack nuts, a digging stick, and a kaross in which to carry them. Three to four days per week

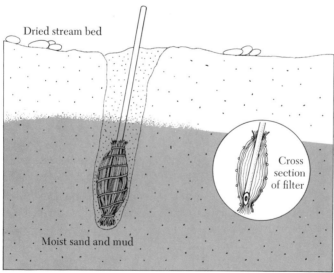

Figure 6-3. Grass filter and tube used by Bushmen for drawing water from below surface of dry stream bed. (After Forde, C. Daryll, *Habitat, Economy and Society*. New York: E. P. Dutton & Co., Inc., 1952.)

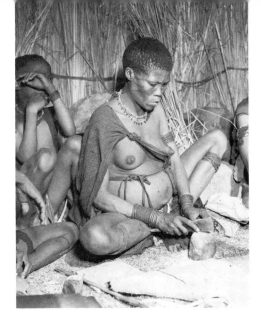

Figure 6-4. Bushwoman forming a bead from an ostrich egg shell. (Courtesy of the South African Information Service.)

were spent in collecting. When nearby groves were exhausted, the women foraged at increasing distances. In wet weather, a band would often change water holes to be closer to a grove, but in the dry season when the bands were restricted to permanent water holes, foraging women often had to travel ten to fifteen miles in a day to reach mongongo trees.

Hunting-gathering technology is often quite ingenious. Some Bushman bands hunt wild fowl by taking advantage of the bird's instinctive behavior patterns. Guinea hens, for example, will attempt instinctively to roll displaced eggs back into their nests. Hunters will remove an egg and place a buried noose about it. The returning hen will roll the egg back to the nest with her beak and be snared by the noose.

Finding water is often a challenge in the dry season. Bushmen will seek out the dried bed of a lake or stream and collect subsurface water with an ingenious sucking tube (Figure 6-3).

Domestic technologies are largely the responsibility of women. Animal skins are fashioned into clothing and bags. The woman's kaross is both a garment and a carry-all. It can be tied at the shoulder and waist in such a way that food, firewood, and perhaps a baby can all be placed in its folds. In addition to gourds, ostrich eggs often serve as containers. Women build the *scherms* or huts which each family occupies. A scherm is typically about four feet high and made of light sticks, twigs, and grass. The floor is covered with grass and a fire pit is built in front of the hut.

In summary, the Bushman's technology, or that of any hunting-gathering group, has these key traits:

1. By our standards, it is extremely simple. The tools a hunter-gatherer uses are handmade and limited in variety. Although often clever, they can be understood readily by any intelligent member of the band, and most of a band's technology can easily be mastered by any one person. The objects fashioned by these tools have the same qualities as the tools themselves.

2. In hunting-gathering technology almost no machines exist to increase the efficiency of daily tasks. The term machine here refers to a device such as an air conditioner or an electric motor which has the ability to take energy from the environment and perform work in the absence of a human hand to guide it. In theory, at least, there are only two limits to a machine's capacity to perform work: the availability of raw materials for it to work on and the availability of fuel to power it. With some exceptions (Figure 6-5), hunting-gathering technology is hand powered and thus can perform less work per person than can our machine technology.

3. The hunter-gatherer's technology is strongly interwoven with his belief in the supernatural.

4. Hunting-gathering technology has a personal quality. Everyone knows who fashioned a certain tool and to whom it belongs.

5. Innovation is rare in hunting-gathering technology, at least in comparison to ours. For example, most of the technology used by a con-

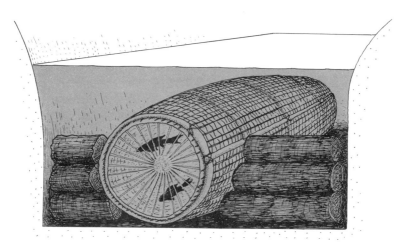

Figure 6-5. Fish trap used by the Kwakiutl Indians of British Columbia. Fish swim into open end of basket and are unable to escape. Is this device a tool or machine or both?

temporary Bushman resembles that of his ancestors. This does not mean the Bushmen are lacking in some key aptitude, for the same conservatism has existed among all hunter-gatherers, including those of prehistoric Europe.

In part, the conservatism of hunting-gathering technology may relate to its association with a belief in the supernatural. Animistic belief systems are authoritarian and have a conservative influence on anything with which they associate. The slowness of change typical of hunter-gatherer technology also seems related to a property inherent in technology itself. In most of the technology that man has developed to date, complexity and innovation seem to be directly related. This, of course, begs the question of which, if either, is the causal factor. We will look again at technological change when we leave hunting-gathering man and turn to Western culture.

6. Hunting-gathering technology is naturalistic. It requires a constant contact with and intimate knowledge of the natural world.

ENVIRONMENT

Generally speaking, hunting-gathering technologies have little impact on the natural environment. There are two reasons for this:

1. Because of his primitive technology, hunting-gathering man must go out into nature to supply his needs. As a result, his population density typically has been low. This must be so, for any undue concentration of people in one region would threaten to exhaust the natural resources he must hunt and gather. Bushman bands, for example, are widely scattered. At least before the advent of Westerners in the region, the Kalahari probably contained less than one Bushman per square mile and a band roamed an area of five hundred to fifteen hundred square miles. As a result, the Bushman's impact on nature is relatively light, and it is possible to travel over the Kalahari for days and see no sign of human life. When some resource, such as the mongongo nuts used by Bushmen, does become depleted, a band will move on, allowing the denuded area to return to normal.

2. The material goods produced by the technology of hunting-gathering man have little impact on the flow of matter within ecosystems. This is partly so because the volume of these goods is so limited. The Bushman, for example, lives in a kind of stable state regarding his material wealth. He is likely to own the same number of pots and arrows at forty as he did, at twenty. Bushman camps are so meager in material wealth that they seem a part of nature. As

Thomas writes: "I once walked right into an empty werf, as their tiny villages are called, and didn't see the little scherms, or huts, hidden in the grass until I noticed a small skin bag dangling in a shadow, which was a doorway." [10]

The objects the Bushman's technology does produce are also easy on ecosystems because they are little altered from their natural state. Clothes are formed directly from skins or plant fibers. If dyed, the dyes are natural. Utensils, houses, and other goods are made of wood, gourds, bone, hide, or sinew. Floors are dirt. Drinking water is untreated; food is without chemical additives. All this means that pollution tends to be minimal. It is true that hunter-gatherers are not particularly sanitary and tend to dump their wastes, whether broken gourds, clay pots, hut saplings, or human waste, into the surrounding environment. Because they are close to their natural state, however, these materials are readily accepted and absorbed back into ecosystems.

A large portion of the hunter-gatherer's day is spent in activities such as dancing, gossiping, or sitting by the fire, activities that we would characterize as leisurely. One study of a Bushman band showed that the band spent only twelve to nineteen hours per week in food-getting activity. Even the most diligent individual in the band spent only thirty-two hours per week in this pursuit.

Why, one might ask, do not Bushmen or other hunter-gatherers increase their work week to forty hours and thus take more from nature and amass more material wealth?

One answer to this is that we are dealing with a circular situation. Hunter-gatherers have a simple, hand-powered technology which forces them to go out into nature for their wants. This in turn leads to a rather meager material wealth, for a nomadic or semi-nomadic band cannot carry much, nor has it the technology to store much of a surplus. Such a band thus lives in a state of limited expectations regarding material goods. With neither need nor place for amassed goods in their life style, why do any more work than that which provides one with food for the next few days or weeks? We tend to think of this lack of concern with growth or with the future as apathetic; to Bushmen it is the normal way of life.

HEALTH

A Bushman's body is the product of a million years of hunting-gathering life. During this time it has become adapted to make him able to cope with all the physical demands this life implies. Consider the demands placed upon the Bushman's heart and skeleton and how each has evolved to meet them.

As a Bushman moves across the Kalahari, his heart must increase its rate in order to supply his body with needed energy. When he runs at top speed, its flow rate must increase eightfold. To meet demands such as these, the Bushman's heart has evolved into a machine more efficient than any man has ever designed. Although it weighs less than a pound, his heart will pump the body's ten pints of blood through a thousand cycles a day. In a seventy-year lifetime, it will pump 600,000 tons of blood, the result of over two billion heartbeats. All of this blood is pushed through a network of arteries, veins, and capillaries—a network at least 60,000 miles in length.

A Bushman's bones are marvelous structures. He has 206, and they range in size from his femur or thighbone—20 inches long and an inch thick, to bones within his wrist that are no larger than a pea. Bone itself is a living tissue, composed of nerves, blood vessels, and cells, all imbedded in a honeycomb of minerals. This porous honeycomb structure is an adaptive response to the powerful force of gravity, for it is both lightweight and very strong. This is of definite survival value when one considers that during the mere act of walking an average Bushman will place up to 1200 pounds per square inch on his thighbone.

As a Bushman strides along, perhaps stalking some game, a series of skeletal adaptations come into play. The arches of his feet absorb the shocks of walking or running while leaving space on the underside of the foot for muscles, blood vessels, and nerves. His pelvis resembles that of his tree-dwelling ancestors, but it is shortened and broadened, adaptations for upright posture. Its new shape provides greater stability and a greater area for attachment of those muscles needed for walking. The flat surfaces of the pelvis also provide support for the overlying organs.

The Bushman's body build is also a result of adaptive pressures of life in the Kalahari climate. The Bushman's body is rather small and lean. A body of this sort tends to have more surface area for its weight than, for example, a squat build such as is associated with the Eskimo. In either case, the build reflects the demands of the local climate. For much of the year, the Kalahari is a hot region, and a body with a high surface-area-to-weight ratio sheds heat more efficiently than a squat build. Some Bushman women have a rather unusual physical condition called *steatopygia*, in which the buttocks are greatly enlarged (Figure 6-6). Most anthropologists believe steatopygia is also

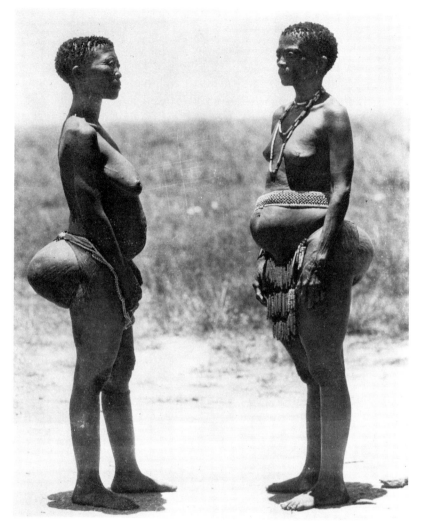

Figure 6-6. Steatopygia.
(Courtesy of the South African Information Service.)

an adaptation to a hot climate, a way to store reserve fat without insulating the whole body.

In his daily life, a Bushman makes full use of his body. Although small of stature and lean of build, Bushmen can carry loads equal to their own weight and are able to travel over the desert for hours on end without visible fatigue. However, the Bushman's superb physical condition is not simply the result of carrying heavy loads. It also comes from the day-to-day punishment associated with a hunting-gathering life. With his scherm, his fire, and a modest array of household goods, the Bushman in his little settlement exists as a part of nature, fully exposed to its hardships. Thomas describes one Bushman camp thus:

> They had burned all their firewood the night before, and now it was too cold to go for more, or even to go for food, so they sat cold, hungry, thirsty, and even tired, since they had been too cold to sleep during the night. They were waiting, as they had waited all night, with infinite patience, infinite endurance, for noonday, when the sun would give a little warmth; but the sky was overcast, and even at noon the sun would still be far away.[11]

Most of us equate this sort of experience with a disastrous camping trip we have had at one time or another. For the Bushman, it is simply a part of living. Going out into nature—roughing it with only a tent and a few implements—can be physically devastating for those accustomed to living in a world of padded chairs and central heating. Eventually, however, the constant exposure to sun, wind, and cold and the continuous physical buffeting, whether from carrying wood or clambering about uneven surfaces or simply sitting on the cold ground, will produce physical tone. This physical tone, which is so sadly lacking among all but a few Americans, is the normal condition for Bushmen and other hunter-gatherers.

The physical condition of hunter-gatherers has not been achieved without cost. Hunter-gatherers appear fit to Westerners in part because weaker or malformed individuals are not in evidence. In hunting-gathering cultures the weeding-out process we call natural selection is in full force, relentlessly eliminating those who fail to measure up physically.

Although famine has certainly been an important selective agent among hunter-gatherers, it has probably not taken as high a toll as might be thought. Typically, hunter-gatherers use a wide range of foodstuffs, so that a shortage of one or two staples can be compensated for by shifting to other foods. Most of the hunting-gathering groups where famine has been an important selective agent have lived in marginal areas—the Eskimos are an example of this.

Some anthropologists feel that warfare was rare or absent among most hunter-gatherers, but research carried out during the last decade among South American Indians suggests that at least there, warfare was an important cause of mortality. If these Indians are at all typical of the primitive situation, aggression between men must have always been an important agent of natural selection.

Disease has certainly been an important selective factor, perhaps the most important one of all. Many studies indicate that hunting-gathering peoples are and probably were not too fastidious about sanitation or personal hygiene. Utensils used in cooking often went unwashed or were used in common. Food or other organic remains sometimes accumulated in and around huts. Bathing, at least in dry regions, was rare. Food sometimes spoiled before it was eaten. Items such as sterile drinking cups, tap water, window screens, soap, a change of clothes, and refrigerators, all of which sever us from the disease microorganisms in our environment, were absent in the hunting-gathering world. As a result, the children of primitives were exposed to disease organisms from an early age. About the South American Xavante and Yanomama, Neel has said that newborn infants "are in an intimate contact with their environment that would horrify a modern mother—or physician. They nurse at sticky breasts, at which the young mammalian pets of the village have also suckled, and soon are crawling on the feces-contaminated soil and chew-

VESTIGES

Most of our body structures seem admirably designed for an active terrestrial existence. There are exceptions, however. Some parts of our body seem to have no purpose. Examples of such parts are the ear muscles—some of us can work these; others cannot—the appendix, and the coccyx or tailbone. Structures such as these are termed *vestigial*. Evolutionary theory explains them as leftovers of a far distant past when these parts had an adaptive role to play. Among arboreal animals a tail plays an important role as a balancing, or sometimes as a grasping, organ. All active animals with good hearing—dogs and cats for example—continually move their outer ears to catch sound more efficiently. Among many herbivorous animals, an appendix has an important role in the digestive process. Since our distant ancestors were probably arboreal, were acutely aware of their surroundings, and were herbivorous, we still carry, in vestigial form, the organs concerned with these activities.

In addition to vestigial structures, we show our evolutionary past in yet another way. Some of our body parts have not as yet become completely redesigned for terrestrial life. They do their job inefficiently, because for them the process of adaptation is incomplete. The pelvic

ing on an unbelievable variety of objects." [12] This sort of exposure produces one dividend. It can build an early and often lifelong tolerance for infectious microorganisms. Significantly, Neel found high levels of gamma globulin, a substance containing generalized antibodies or proteins which defend against infection, among Yanomama children. On the other hand, many young children must have succumbed to childhood infections, particularly of the gastrointestinal tract, which were a result of these unsanitary conditions.

Before contact with Western civilization, contagious diseases such as influenza or measles were almost certainly absent, for they need large, dense aggregates of people in order to flourish. Cancer and cardiovascular disease were also unusual among hunter-gatherers. To judge from evidence provided by skeletal remains, some of the degenerative diseases, particularly bone pathology, may not have been uncommon, and hunting-gathering man apparently had his arthritis problems just as we do!

Accidents certainly took their toll. Injuries from falls must have been

opening is a good example of such a structure. The frequency of Caesarean operations attests to the fact that the pelvic opening has not yet become large enough to accomodate the large-brained babies produced by modern man. Several parts of the skeleton have failed to keep up with man's evolution toward a bipedal life style. The backbone is a well-known example. Although a remarkable structure, it still suffers from faulty design, as indicated by the frequency of lower back ailments and slipped discs. The sinuses also are obsolete in their design. They are built to drain toward the front of the head. The system worked well when we moved about on all fours, but it does not work so well now, and infected sinuses are the price we pay for this evolutionary lag. Finally, the circulatory system has not kept complete pace with our shift to a terrestrial existence. No other mammals faint. Man does so because his circulatory system has not developed quite enough pressure to keep his head supplied with blood during certain kinds of stress situations. At the other end of our body, hemorrhoids and varicose veins in the legs are the consequences of a blood pressure which is greater than that region of the circulatory system was designed to handle.

common. Special hazards existed, dependent on local conditions. Drowning, for example, is common among the Eskimo, while eye injuries from branches are common among the Bushmen.

Among hunting-gathering peoples the sick and injured are tended by medicine men. These are band members who practice medicine as a task added to their usual activities. Although some herbs may be used which seem to have medicinal value, most of a medicine man's effectiveness stems from his powers of suggestion over the patient. Since sickness is thought to result from the invasion of spirits into the body, *object removal* is a common treatment. After various preliminary exhortations, the medicine man finally locates an object in the patient, which is identified as the source of trouble. The object—a bit of bark or stone which the medicine man had earlier hidden on his person—is

PHYSIOLOGICAL ADAPTABILITY

Although our body structure and function are under genetic control, genes provide only the broadest of instructions. Much of the physical variation that we see between one person and another is not genetic at all, but a result of nongenetic physiological adaptation to the environment.

As suggested in the text, a person can develop either a hardened body or a soft, fat one. The difference is dependent upon his life style, not on his genes, for the latter remain the same regardless of his physical condition. Some other examples of physiological adaptation follow.

1. Biological rhythms. A number of metabolic activities in the human body operate in cycles. Some of these cycles are *circadian,* that is, they have a twenty-four-hour period. Some have a cycle which approximates the lunar period. Rhythms such as these have been demonstrated for our red blood cell count, the amount of sugar and iron in the body, for adrenaline activity, and many other metabolic variables. Many of our bodily mechanisms seem to slow during the night, then pick up just before dawn. Although these rhythms presumably have a genetic base, they can be adjusted to new environments. We do not yet know enough about the body's rhythms to tell just what the biological cost of a readjustment is. However, as anyone who has flown across time zones knows, the readjustment of these rhythms can be an uncomfortable process.

2. Changes in climate. A northerner who moves to Florida in sum-

removed and the patient pronounced well. Although this is merely sleight of hand to us, to a believing patient the treatment probably has definite psychological value. Among some groups, *trephination* was practiced. This painful operation, which involved opening the skull, may have had some utility in relieving fractures but probably killed more often than it cured.

The generally ineffective medical technology of hunting-gathering peoples implies that among them disease and accident have probably always acted as powerful agents of selection, removing those who were weaker or in some way prone to illness or accident.

In addition to extrinsic agents of natural selection such as famine, predation, and disease, hunting-gathering peoples have commonly utilized intrinsic self-regulating agents. These have had the dual func-

mertime is likely to find the climate of his new home almost unbearably hot and sticky. After a few weeks or months, however, he becomes used to it. In contrast, southerners find a New England winter impossibly cold. They also will become acclimated. In either case, the adjustment is physiological. In effect, the body learns to match its climate-control mechanisms to the new environment.

3. Long-range physiological adaptation. Some physiological adaptations begin at birth. Adaptations of this type are likely to have a greater effect on the body's structure and function than the short-range adjustments we mentioned above. Americans mature earlier and are taller than their great-grandfathers. Some of this change may be genetic, but most of it is probably a physiological adaptation to a better diet and better living conditions.

4. Adjustment to a completely new environment. After their long stays in space, the Skylab astronauts were found to have lost significant amounts of muscle tissue, calcium, and red blood cells. The loss of calcium and muscle tissue was apparently a physiological adaptation to weightlessness. Blood cells decreased because the spacemen breathed an atmosphere with a higher oxygen content than is found on earth and thus needed fewer red blood cells, which transport oxygen to the lungs. In this respect it is interesting to note that Peruvian Indians of the Andes Mountains have more red blood cells than is average, an adaptation to the oxygen-poor air of high altitudes.

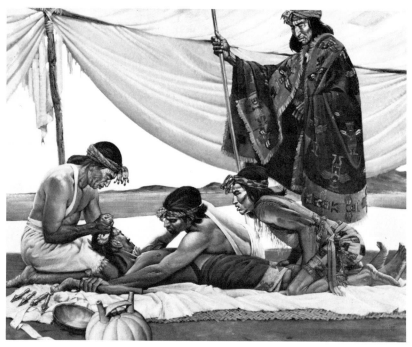

Figure 6-7. Trephination in ancient Peru. (Courtesy of Parke, Davis & Company © 1957.)

tion of weeding out the weak or unfit and maintaining the population on a more or less stable level. One common self-regulating practice is infanticide. Among many Bushman bands, babies are not weaned for three or four years. This has a contraceptive effect on the mother, but only a partial one. Should she become pregnant before the earlier child is weaned or when the band is short of food, a mother may have to kill her newborn. This unpleasant task is usually carried out by an older woman rather than by the mother herself. While a Bushman mother may anguish over her loss, the demands of band survival permit her no choice. In addition, deformed or sickly children are killed in many groups. Estimates have ranged from fifteen to fifty per cent respecting the average infanticide rate among hunting-gathering peoples.

On rare occasions, elderly people may be abandoned to die if drought and scarcity force the group to seek new territory and it is obvious that some elderly person will not be able to keep up with the band.

PRESENT
PART II

We will begin Part II by asking why a new kind of technology, which we will call Western, has come to dominate the world. Two events—domestication and the rise of that view of reality we call *scientific*—seem to us the crucial events which acted to open the way for the rise of Western technology. After a look at each of these, we will examine Western technology itself. Finally, we will analyze the impact of the new technology, first on the natural environment and then on the health of man himself.

7

DOMESTICATION

As we have seen through our examination of the Bushmen, hunting-gathering cultures generally had relatively little impact on the natural environment. As does any generalization, however, this statement needs to be qualified. We will look at two exceptions to this statement, since they foreshadowed what was to come.

A variety of large plant-eating mammals, including the mammoth, mastodon, wooly rhinoceros, giant sloth, and Irish elk, became extinct between ten and fifty thousand years ago. Paleontologists have long puzzled over this. At one time, many thought the ice ages were responsible. Better data, however, seem to indicate that these extinctions were not correlated with any change in climate. What could have been involved? One cause-and-effect relationship stands out above all others. As shown in Figure 7-1, there seems to have been a direct correlation between the spread of hunting-gathering man across the globe and the sequence in which animal extinction took place. Although the correlation is an intriguing one, the issue of whether it is real has not been settled. If prehistoric hunter-gatherers did indeed exterminate large numbers of species, this would suggest that even before the rise of domestication man's technology had enough power to begin the long process of disruption which has culminated in today's environmental crisis.

Although most hunter-gatherers have lived in a state of limited ex-

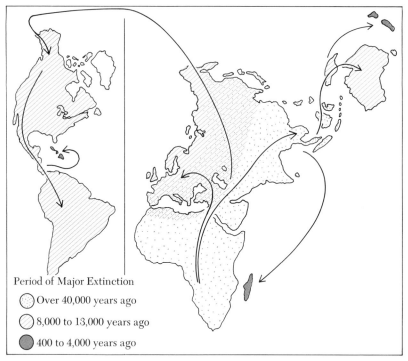

Figure 7-1. Global pattern of prehistoric faunal extinction. Arrows indicate migrations of early man from presumed origin in Africa.

pectations respecting material goods, not all have done so. In some parts of the world the environment has been rich enough so that even a hunting-gathering technology could produce an affluent society. Our northwest coast from Alaska to northern California is an example of such an environment. The climate is wet but mild. Natural resources abound. The area, at least before the white man's occupancy, was unbelievably rich in sea life. Tall forests of spruce, hemlock, and cedar crowded down to the shore. Elk, moose, and deer were common. A number of Indian tribes, of which the best known were the Tlingit, Haida, and Kwakiutl, lived along this lush coast. The life of each tribe was centered in a semipermanent village made up of a long row of wooden houses which faced the water (Figure 7-2). Each house was a massive and elaborate structure. Built of wood, it housed several families and could be a hundred feet or more in length. During the leisurely winter months, tribesmen occupied this village, repairing tools, canoes, or other equipment. During spring and summer temporary fishing and collecting camps were established. With the aid of nets, harpoons, and traps, northwest coast hunters accumulated large stores of fish. Forest game was generally neglected, except for that needed to provide wool, skin, horn, or sinew. The fish, along with a rich harvest of berries and roots, were preserved for the winter months. This more than ample subsistence base and the sedentary life which accompanied it allowed the northwest coast Indians to develop an impressive material culture. Indian craftsmen fashioned elaborate objects of wood, copper, bone, and stone. Some families came to have noble status and owned the rights to fishing and collecting grounds; some kept captives taken in war as slaves. Rather elaborate rules of inheritance developed. Above all, the *potlatch feasts* were symbolic of the material wealth developed by northwest coast Indians. A noble family would give one of these feasts and invite other nobles, who would be seated according to their status. A kind of giveaway orgy followed, in which the host showered his guests with all manner of

Figure 7-2. Northwest coast Indian village; photograph probably taken in late 19th century. Clothing and signs on houses reflect Western influence. (Courtesy of the American Museum of Natural History.)

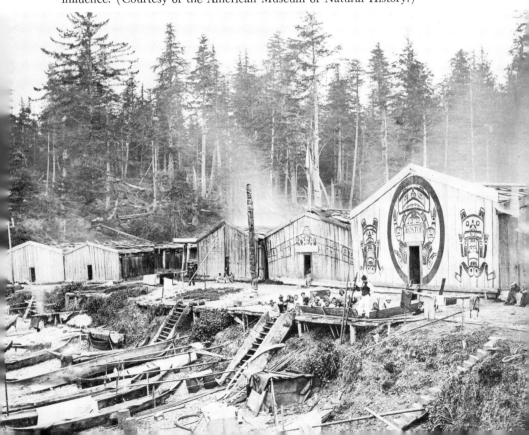

gifts. Those nobles who gave the best and the most at their feasts had highest status and—shades of the future—nobles would sometimes go into debt to prepare a feast which exceeded the efforts of their peers.

In spite of long-range environmental changes such as extinction of fauna and in spite of local areas of material affluence such as the northwest coast, most of the hunting-gathering people lived more in the style of the Bushmen. Their life was not to change until the arrival of that new technology we call domestication.

Where, why, and when did men first domesticate wild plants and animals? This probably happened independently at several different times and in several different regions. We will concentrate on events in the Near East, since the domestication which arose there formed a base for the subsequent rise of Western technology.

Almost all authorities on the subject agree that in the Near East domestication arose along the so-called Fertile Crescent. In the millenia which preceded domestication, the foothills bordering this area harbored wild forms of wheat, barley, lentils, and peas. Wild sheep, goats, pigs, and cattle were also common in the region. Archaeological evidence indicates that sometime around 10,000 B.C. hunting-gathering groups had settled in semipermanent camps or villages among these hills and had begun the long process of domestication.

The first evidence of domestication in the area comes from some

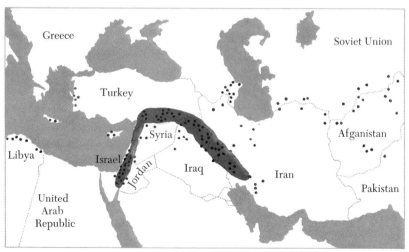

Figure 7-3. Domestication of barley and wheat. Dots indicate probable location of wild grasses; dark crescent, the region where domestication probably took place.

open-air encampments in northeastern Iraq which have yielded eleven-thousand-year-old bones identified as those of domestic sheep. This conclusion is based both on the structure of the bones and the fact that about sixty per cent of them are from yearlings, an indication that the camp occupants were husbanding sheep and selectively slaughtering the young animals for food. The oldest evidence for plant domestication also comes from village sites in Iraq and dates to about nine thousand years ago.

How and why did domestication begin in the Near East?

One view sees plant domestication as a kind of gradual, unconscious process associated with collecting activity. Sickles, mortars, and caches of wild cereal grains are found in some early village sites, suggesting an intensive collection of wild grains. Experiments have shown that one person could have collected more than four pounds of grain an hour using a primitive flint sickle. Grain collected in the foothill regions would be brought back to the villages, where some would be accidentally dropped and would take root in the cleared areas surrounding each village. Gradually, villagers would come purposefully to plant some of the grain they collected. Those plants with the most desirable characteristics would be favored, leading to a slow selection for those characteristics we associate with domestic grains.

Another view sees plant domestication as less of an accidental process and more the result of a policy decision. According to this view, in some areas overcrowding forced hunting-gathering peoples to migrate to less favored regions. Those who were forced to leave would decide to take some of the abundant wild grains with them and would deliberately plant these in their new homeland, thus beginning the practice of agriculture.

Just as with plants, no one really knows how or why the first animals were domesticated. Young sheep and calves may first have been kept as pets. Older animals, particularly wild cattle, may have been initially captured in connection with religious fertility rites. Once domesticated, both sheep and cattle were probably raised for their meat. Only after thousands of years of breeding would the milk cows and wool-bearing sheep with which we are familiar appear.

Domestication brought a series of social and technological changes of the greatest significance. Collectively these opened the way for the rise of modern Western technology. In summary form, these changes were as follows:

1. *Development of a surplus.* No longer were men forced to go out into nature for their needs. Instead, agricultural man could take

Kilocalories in Thousands

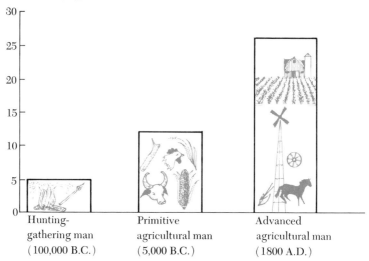

Figure 7-4. With only energy from fire and the food he ate, primitive man used about 5,000 kilocalories a day. Early agricultural man, with his crops and animal power, used 12,000. Advanced agricultural man, with access to machinery, used 26,000 kilocalories a day. Figures are approximate. (Data from Cook, Carl, "The Flow of Energy in an Industrial Society," *Scientific American,* 224, September 1971, pp. 135–144.)

selected species into his own domain and manage these in order to produce the greatest possible return.

It is obviously more efficient to have one's plant food concentrated in neat rows than scattered through miles of savannah. In the same way, it takes much less energy to harvest meat from a flock or herd within a compound than to stalk it through the forest. Later, when primitive ox-drawn plows came into use, this efficiency was increased still further, for manpower became augmented by oxen power. Domestication thus increased the work energy available to each man, as shown in Figure 7-4.

The greater efficiency and the resultant ability to gather more from nature per man-hour than hunter-gatherers ever could led to the possibility of accumulating a surplus, that is, taking more from nature than was necessary for mere subsistence.

2. *A sedentary life.* Some agriculturalists continued to follow a semi-nomadic existence, as did those groups who came to specialize in the herding of animals. Most agriculturalists, however, abandoned the old migratory ways and settled in one place, there to tend and watch their crops. Many of us think of a farming life as a solitary one. Through most of history, however, farmers have been villagers. The first Near

Eastern farmers and those of Europe who followed lived together in villages and walked or rode out to their crops. In some regions, especially in the Near East, the Orient, and the New World, a well-organized, highly efficient agricultural base produced pre-industrial cities. Basically, these cities were clusters of farming villages grouped about a ceremonial and ruling center. Sedentary life, whether in village or city, led to a great increase in worldliness. A typical villager would have impressed us as naive and limited in his ideas; yet he was more sophisticated than his hunting-gathering ancestors had ever been. He was in daily contact with more people and, as we suggest in the next paragraph, with people of increasingly divergent skills. The citizen of a pre-industrial city would be much more exposed to a cosmopolitan environment than his country cousin.

3. *The rise of specialists.* Since agriculture could provide a surplus, this meant that not all villagers were needed to provide the community with its subsistence base. Gradually, a small group of specialists arose who spent little if any time in food production but instead provided the village with other services. This pattern had

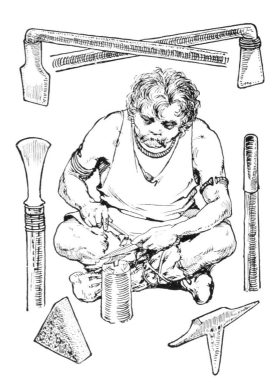

Figure 7-5. A smith of the primitive agricultural era surrounded by his tools. On top are his hammers; to the left a tonged chisel; to the right a socketed gouge; and underneath a sandstone and a simple anvil. (Courtesy of the American Museum of Natural History.)

begun to develop among the wealthier hunting-gathering cultures, such as those of the northwest coast; now it became the norm rather than the exception. Artisans, priests, even soldier classes arose, particularly in the more advanced agricultural societies.

4. *The rise of machine power.* Agriculture is a two-way commitment. It produces material wealth for its practitioner, but in order to gain this wealth, he must successfully tend and harvest his crops and herds. To a degree, this can be done by hand or, even better, done with the aid of animal power. Ultimately, however, it becomes desirable for additional sources of power to be found to thresh the grain, fill the irrigation ditches, and do all the other tasks associated with domestication. With the rise of the specialist artisan class that always accompanies advanced agriculture, a further need for power is created, for a metal worker or potter needs power to aid him in turning his potter's wheel or heating his forge. The new kind of agricultural society thus came to develop machines of increasing power and complexity (Figure 7-6).

5. *The move away from nature.* Hunting-gathering man had no choice; his methods of subsistence forced him to live within nature. Although agricultural man was still very much aware of his natural environment, his life style marked the beginning of a new era. Even the humblest of agricultural villages is different from the Bushman camp, for agricultural man has begun the long process of fencing out nature.

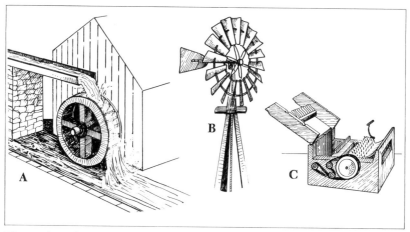

Figure 7-6. Three machines used by agricultural man: A. water wheel; B. windmill; C. cotton gin.

Agricultural man's relationship with nature undergoes other changes. His numbers increase, thus greatly accelerating that imbalance between man and other species which was foreshadowed in hunting-gathering man's pressure on the large herbivores he hunted. Man's activity as a pollutor now becomes much more evident. Unlike his nomadic ancestors, the sedentary agriculturalist could not outrun his wastes, and often they accumulated in great masses around and within his villages.

6. *A new way of viewing nature.* In many areas of the world, including the Near East, water is a problem. Successful agriculture requires the development of irrigation to supplement the scant annual rainfall. These areas developed so-called *hydraulic civilizations,* agricultures based upon highly complex irrigation systems. The hydraulic civilizations which arose in the Near East, China, India, and certain areas of the New World were the originators of what we call civilization—that is, they were the agricultural societies which gave rise to cities, writing, and ultimately to science. The sophistication of hydraulic civilizations was gained at a price. The elaborate irrigation systems were maintained by armies of peasants, who were required to devote part of their time to maintenance work. For a sophisticated irrigation system to work successfully, it was necessary to predict annual changes in rainfall and other natural phenomena of importance to agriculture. Thus, the priests of hydraulic civilizations became increasingly involved in the study of natural phenomena and became particularly adept in astronomy. Although their explanations of events such as eclipses or phases of the moon were still animistic, the techniques they developed to study these events and the data they collected were to form the base for a new and different view of reality, which we will examine in the next chapter.

8

There are two ways of defining science, each of equal importance. First, science is a particular view of what nature is like. Second, science is a particular view about how we can best come to know and understand nature.

WHAT NATURE IS LIKE

To the Catholic Church of medieval Europe, the universe was a great sphere, built of concentric crystalline layers or shells, rather like an onion. The motionless earth lay at the center of this universe. The earth, home of mortal man, was made of four elements—earth, air, fire, and water. Of these, fire was the purest and noblest, earth the meanest element. Each element possessed an urge to attain its rightful place in the scheme of things. Earth, as the basest element, strove to fall inward toward hell; fire, as the noblest element, pushed outward toward the heavens surrounding the earth. If the elements achieved their rightful positions, the world would then be made of four layers, earth, water, air, and fire. The earth then would be still and content, for each element would have finally found its rightful place. The Catholic churchmen believed this could never happen because the elements of the world were too mixed. The result of this mixing was the unstable, unpredictable, and imperfect condition of things which they saw about them. To the churchmen, the shells beyond the earth were made of a glassy crystal-line ether—invisible, yet with enough consistency to support the planets, sun, and stars. Except for that one which contained the moon, the heavenly shells beyond the earth were seen as incorruptible and perfect. The shell containing the moon was thought of as having not yet attained a state of perfection. This imperfection was evident, for, unlike other heavenly bodies, the moon was blemished. These heavenly shells were thought to move in a circular path, for only this kind of motion was considered perfect. The eighth shell out contained the stars; the ninth, just beyond it, was the *primum mobile*. This shell, the prime mover, turned itself and all inner shells. Its motion was ardent, for just beyond it lay the Empyrean Heaven, home of God.

The medieval universe was seen in holistic terms. It was a coherent universe, in which everything had a role to play and strove to achieve its particular purpose in the larger scheme of things. As seen by medieval churchmen the universe was under the control of a host of beings. God himself was both the creator and continuing ruler of the universe. Bands of angels—the Seraphim, Cherubim, and others—ran the heavenly shells. Lucifer, a deposed angel, ran Hell. Just as man was subordinate to this host of spiritual beings, nature was sub-ordinate to man and designed to serve his ends. It was a personalized universe, filled with and run by individual beings rather than natural laws. To the medieval churchmen the universe and all reality were purposeful. Man was destined to follow a divinely ordained progres-sion from creation to final union with God. The medieval universe thus was animistic. Although this universe had a kind of awesome grandeur to it, it was nevertheless a human universe, with subjective, emo-tional, human characteristics such as fear, love, and hope, char-acteristics with which the common man could relate. It is symbolic of this animistic, human universe that its best description is not to be found in some learned treatise, but in Dante's *Divine Comedy,* that great epic poem of man's progression to paradise (Figure 8-1A).

Just as did the medieval churchman, the modern scientist sees order in the universe, but beyond this all resemblance stops. Figure 8-1B depicts the Hertzsprung-Russell diagram, which plots the absolute visual magnitudes of stars against their spectra. The stars shown are from the Hyades cluster. In contrast to the medieval churchman's holistic view of the universe, the Hertzsprung-Russell diagram is re-ductionistic. Rather than attempting to construct a complete image of the universe, it deals with only one set of objects—the stars—and one set of phenomena—their spectra and absolute visual magnitude

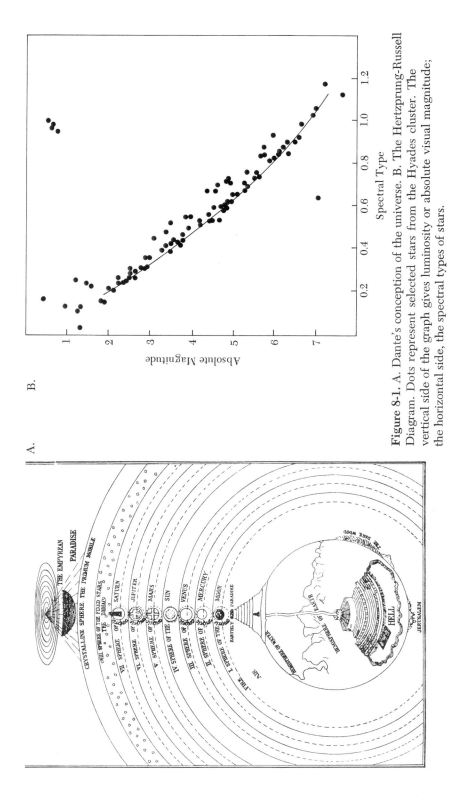

Figure 8-1. A. Dante's conception of the universe. B. The Hertzsprung-Russell Diagram. Dots represent selected stars from the Hyades cluster. The vertical side of the graph gives luminosity or absolute visual magnitude; the horizontal side, the spectral types of stars.

or luminosity. While the scientist has as his ultimate aim a holistic image of reality, he commonly works with one piece of it at a time.

The medieval churchman saw a purposeful universe which operated according to the designs of God. As far as the scientist is concerned there may be such a purpose, but its existence is outside the realm of scientific exploration. No angels can be found in the Hertzsprung-Russell diagram. What the scientist sees is a lawfulness which can be described mathematically, a rather precise relationship between star spectra and star luminosity. From this he can derive a formula, that is, a relationship expressed in mathematical terms. Using this formula he can predict the spectra of some new star if he has information about its luminosity. What this relationship means, that is, whether the relationship is indicative of some larger purpose in nature, is beyond his interest as a scientist.

HOW AND WHAT WE CAN KNOW OF REALITY

When the medieval church built its picture of the universe, it peopled this universe with objects drawn from everyday life. In contrast, since scientific images of the universe are built upon mathematical symbols which are not drawn from everyday life, they are

REALITY AS SEEN BY ART AND BY SCIENCE

In his book *The Tao of Science* R.G.H. Siu has this to say about art and science:

"Poetic language induces a mood. We observe its charm in a poem, a symphony, a painting, a ballet. It stresses the quality of emotions rather than the utility of experience. The difference between descriptive and poetic language can be illustrated by Eddington's example: If we are concerned with the formation of waves by winds in the physics laboratory, we had best look up the standard descriptive hydrodynamic equations beginning with

$$\frac{p'_{yy}}{g\rho\eta} = \frac{(\alpha^2 + 2\nu k\alpha + \sigma^2)A - i(\sigma^2 + 2\nu km\alpha)C}{gk(A - iC)}$$

"The series of equations goes on to show that winds of less than half a mile an hour leave the surface of the water unruffled. As the speed rises to a mile an hour, minute corrugations appear. Finally, gravity

often unintelligible. Most of us would recognize the Hertzsprung-Russell diagram as a form of graph, but *absolute magnitude* or *spectral type* baffle most of us. The universe described by medieval churchmen was full of unique personalities. The scientist, in contrast, is not as interested in the uniqueness of each star he studies as in the properties they hold in common. With the exception of spectra and magnitude, all of the individual idiosyncrasies of the stars in Figure 8-1B have been smoothed over, and they have become standardized into dots. The scientist thus tries to work with generalized, standardized, quantified phenomena, rather than with unique events.

Just how does the scientist develop his ideas and how does his method compare with that of the medieval churchman? In a very real sense the latter did not develop ideas at all. Medieval churchmen did discuss problems of interpreting reality, but always they came back to an unchanging reference point—the authority which stemmed from church dogma. Thus their answer to the question, "How and what can we know of reality?" was "Seek your answers through the Bible, through revelation, through the Church Fathers." Theirs was an authoritarian, traditionalist view of the way to knowledge. In contrast, scientific concepts are developed and modified through an unending process of exploration we call the *scientific method*.

waves are produced at wind speeds of two miles an hour. Yet were we strolling along the shore, the same thought of the generation of waves by winds might evoke sentiments much more aptly described by Rupert Brooke:

> There are waters blown by changing winds to laughter
> And lit by the rich skies all day and after
>   Frost with a gesture stays the waves that dance,
> And wandering loneliness; he leaves a white
>   Unbroken glory, a gathered radiance,
> A width, a shining peace, under the night." [13]

Is the artist's view of reality the same as that of the medieval churchman? If not, how do their views differ? How would you compare the artist's view, as represented by Brooke's poem, with that of the scientist, represented by the hydrodynamic equation?

THE SCIENTIFIC METHOD

The method that scientists use in their exploration of reality is based on certain assumptions about reality. First, a scientist assumes that some degree of order or pattern is present in nature. By this he means two things: (1) He believes that things in nature do not exist in a completely random fashion, but can be assorted into classes. Any scientist, for example, who studies meteorology will come to see that clouds can be grouped into certain classes with regard to their structure and behavior, or that the event we call a hurricane has certain characteristics common to all hurricanes. In part, these classes are creations of the scientist's mind, but in large part they seem to actually exist in the reality which is assumed to exist apart from our minds. (2) A scientist believes that things and events do not just happen through some divine fiat. They come about through prior causes. If one has enough information and enough insight, it is possible to discover these patterns of cause and effect. To use meteorology again as an example, scientists have discovered that it can be predicted that certain cloud formations, when coupled with other meteorological phenomena, will produce hurricanes. Sometimes these cause-effect networks are rather easily discovered. More often than not, however, scientists must sort out a tangled mass of events and make guesses as to which event is cause and which is effect. Often the events themselves are inferred, not directly perceived. No one has ever seen atoms, yet all of chemistry is based on a belief in their existence.

Scientific work can take many directions. A museum worker may spend his life working with a single group of beetles, learning their relationships and characteristics. A physicist may labor years to define a single cause-effect sequence which will then become one more law of physics. On occasion, much larger syntheses are made. Through exceptional insight many classes of things and events are seen to be causally connected and an atomic theory or a theory of evolution is born.

How do scientists build their images of nature? Whether these are grand theories or modest laws, a common battery of techniques is usually involved. The major components of this technique are:

1. *Observation.* If there is any ultimate authority in science, it is that which can be perceived, either directly via the unaided senses or indirectly via instrumentation. Whatever else he does, a scientist is bound by his peers to respect the observable. In collecting data or

information, he must be as accurate as his senses or the instruments extending his senses will permit. While a scientist does not necessarily begin his work by making observations, the ideas he formulates about patterns in nature inevitably draw upon earlier observations and will be tested by later ones.

2. *Hypothesis.* No scientist runs about recording every bit of information provided by his senses, for the result would be a huge mass of meaningless data. Instead, he works from an initial hypothesis, a hunch or sudden insight concerning a suspected pattern in nature. An hypothesis may be quite specific. A mathematician may suddenly come to suspect that a specific equation may explain some phenomenon in nature. On the other hand, an hypothesis may be no more than a feeling about where to look next or what kind of data might be significant. Such insights may be quite limited or they may be grand schemes which involve a large number of observables.

Where do hypotheses come from? There is no concrete answer to this question—the creation of new ideas is a little-understood process. The concept of natural selection, discussed earlier in this text, provides an example of how new hypotheses arise. Two famous naturalists, Charles Darwin and Alfred Russel Wallace, developed the idea of natural selection independently. In Darwin's case, one can go back through his notebooks and by hindsight pick out all the bits and pieces of information, whether they were ideas gleaned from other workers or observations made by Darwin himself, that provided the raw material from which he built his hypothesis of natural selection. In Wallace's case the idea of natural selection came more abruptly, at a time, incidentally, when the naturalist was suffering from a tropical fever!

3. *Testing.* The 1860's were a time of ferment in medical science. New observations, particularly those which came about through the use of the microscope, were producing fresh insights into the causes of disease. One of these insights was a then-revolutionary hypothesis called the germ theory of disease, which stated that most diseases result from attack by some sort of microorganism. Robert Koch was one of the creators of this hypothesis and one of the first to test its validity. His studies of anthrax, a disease found in sheep, provide a good example of how a scientist goes about testing an hypothesis. First, Koch examined the tissues of sheep with anthrax. In them he identified a suspicious bacterialike agent. Next he managed to isolate and grow the agent and inoculate healthy sheep with it. He then

watched the inoculated animals for any sign of disease. As he predicted, the inoculated sheep contracted anthrax. Again as he predicted, Koch was able to recover the same agent from their diseased tissue. In this way he validated the hypothesis that a microorganism was the cause of anthrax. But if the germ theory were to have a more general validity, that is, if it were to apply to disease in general rather than just to anthrax, one would expect to find infectious agents in a

THE CHILD'S PERCEPTION OF REALITY

The great Swiss psychologist Jean Piaget has spent his professional life seeking to understand how a young child perceives reality and how his perception changes with growth. Here are some examples of his findings.

1. Young children lack the ability to establish what we might call logical cause-and-effect hypotheses.
   Example: Piaget quotes a child who said, "The moon doesn't fall down because there is no sun because it is very high up."
2. Young children lack *conservation.* By this term Piaget means a type of abstraction crucial to science—the ability to realize that certain basic characteristics of an object remain constant regardless of superficial changes in appearance.
   Example: If a very young child is shown two rows of buttons, thus O O O O O O and OOOOOO, he will say the shorter row has fewer buttons than the longer one.
3. Young children lack another sort of ability to abstract, again one which is crucial to science. They cannot separate their own subjective values from objective reality. Their concept of temporal sequences, for example, is typically modified by their own feelings about things.
   Example: A small boy, age four years, nine months, is being questioned about his brothers:

"I have two brothers, Philippe and Robert."
"Are they older or younger than you?"
"Older than me."
"Much older?"
"Yes."
"How old are they?"

variety of diseased tissues. In the 1870's and 1880's, investigations of a variety of human diseases bore out this prediction. As a result of these investigations, the germ theory became generally accepted.

The scientific method is thus a mixture of activities. Any one investigation may start with some hunch or hypothesis which has been developed to account for certain observable facts. This hypothesis will be tested by experiment or by gathering still more data. If it stands up

"I don't know."

"Do they go to the big school?"

"Yes, both of them."

"Is one older than the other?"

"No, both of them are the same age." (*Wrong.*)

"Were they born on the same day?"

"Yes." (*Wrong.*)

"Are they twins?"

"No."

"But they are the same age all the same?"

"Yes, the same age as myself."

"Who was born first then?"

"Philippe and then Robert." (*Correct*)

"Who was born first, Philippe or you?"

"I." (*Wrong.*)

"So who is the oldest of you three?"

"Nobody."

"You told me you were born before Philippe, so you must have been there when Philippe was born?"

"Oh sure, I was there." (*This seemed quite evident to him.*)

"Who was born first in your whole family?"

"No one. Philippe came second, then Robert, and I was the fourth because I am four years old." [14]

4. Finally, young children are animistic. Much as did primitive man, they see all manner of things in their environment as alive and acting with purpose.

Does all this mean that the nonscientific view of reality is infantile, whereas science represents an adult view?

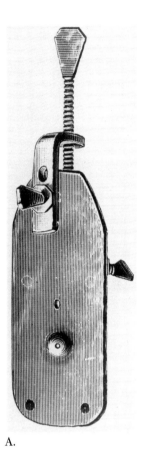

A.

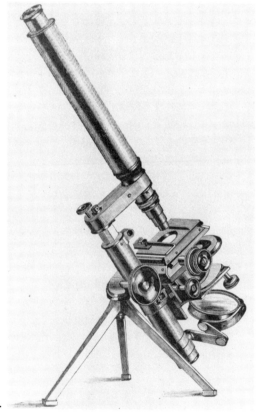

Figure 8-2. Advances in the technology of microscope construction were necessary before major advances could be made in the understanding of infectious disease. A. Primitive hand microscope used by Anthony Leeuwenhoek circa 1700. B. An English microscope of the 1860's.

B.

to these tests, the hypothesis will be accepted as a valid explanation of the observable facts, but only until a better hypothesis is put forth. Because of this, no hypothesis or theory about the order in nature is ever final. In general, those hypotheses which are simpler, which bring together a larger range of observables, and which have a greater ability to predict future events are chosen over competing hypotheses which are weaker in these qualities.

The excitement which accompanies scientific work is perhaps the greatest attraction that science holds for its practitioners. As one writer has put it:

> Anyone who has brought up a bright child is moved and impressed by its insatiable desire to know and to understand the world, to find connections between things and events, a need which most adults no longer seem to have. . . . Science is the survival in mankind of this questing energy of the young, and scientists are the Peter Pans of our culture, the part that does not become indifferent, blasé and tired.[15]

Do the images of nature created by the scientist have a deeper validity than those produced through other means? After all, most religions have had an aim similar to that of science, to create a picture of order from the apparent chaos of nature. The difference between scientific order and religious order lies in one word: predictability. An image of nature as created through religious inspiration may have beauty and meaning, but it lacks the day-to-day utility which is implied by the concept of predictability. In spite of claims to the contrary, no religious view of nature has the power to foretell, to predict in a specific sense, how future events will unfold. In contrast, scientific images of the order which exists in nature do have just this property. The laws which govern the movements of objects in space allow us to say how objects once moved and acted in times past, how they now act, and how they will act in the future. We are confident enough of the predictive power of these laws to stake lives on them, which is just what was done with the astronauts.

Not all scientific images of nature have the same degree of predictability. Those of the physical sciences are typically most exact, those of the biological sciences less so, and those within the social sciences the least. This is due in part to the greater complexity of the types of life and the events with which the social scientist must deal.

9 THE RISE OF WESTERN TECHNOLOGY

Recall our earlier definition of technology as those methods which a culture employs to take things from nature and turn them into useful material objects. How, then, does modern Western technology differ from the technology of other cultures such as the Bushman's? The answer is basically this: Our technology is built on science as a belief system, while the Bushman's technology is built upon animism. This does not mean that Bushmen never experiment with new ways of doing things, but it does mean that within their technology this kind of activity is relatively rare.

Since the natural world of the Bushman is under the control of spirits, it is open to little manipulation or change by man. Things are what they are; experimentation and innovation tend to be discouraged. In contrast, the scientific view of reality leads to a technology which orients itself to experimentation, discovery, change.

Not all nonscientific technologies are as closely associated with animism as the Bushman's is. Medieval Europe developed an empirical trial-and-error technology which was centered neither on animism nor science and which managed to grow lustily and produce quite sophisticated machinery (Figure 9-1). Much of this technology was the work of skilled but illiterate artisans who worked in complete ignorance of the scientific methodologies just then being developed among Europe's learned classes. In spite of the accomplishments of these

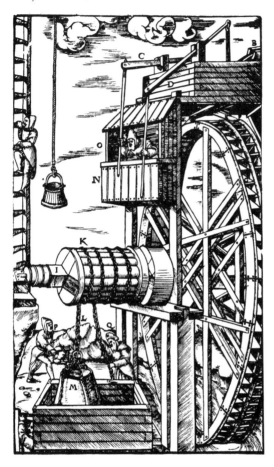

Figure 9-1. A wheel for raising water. (From Agricola, Georgius, *De re Metallica*, Basle, 1556.)

artisans, the modern Western technology of today with its great sophistication and even greater power, would never have developed if this earlier technology had remained independent of science. It was the marriage of the two in Renaissance and post-Renaissance Europe which set the stage for the modern technological world.

THE STEP TO MODERN TECHNOLOGY

The rise of modern Western technology was associated with the larger cultural movement called the Renaissance. During the Renaissance, the older medieval life style, marked by an emphasis on other-worldliness, self-denial, and mysticism, was replaced by a renewed interest in the power of man's body and mind. New forms of art appeared, new lands were discovered, and a new economy based on capitalism arose.

Just what happened in Renaissance Europe to set the stage for modern technology? Many characteristics of Renaissance Europe have been implicated; we will now examine several of these.

1. *Cooperation between natural philosopher and artisan.* The Renaissance philosophers who began to shift Europe away from medieval scholasticism and toward science were often more comfortable with artisans than with the traditional scholars of the universities. Most of the new breed of natural philosophers were either outside the university establishment, or, as in the case of Galileo, came into conflict with it. In the view of traditional scholars, these new philosophers were actually nothing of the kind. Galileo, for example, was regarded as more of a technician than a philosopher. Subjects such as mathematics and even the fine arts which interested the new philosophers were regarded by the traditionalists as not worthy of the interest of true philosophy. Many of the new natural philosophers actually were more technicians than thinkers, for they were interested in working with nature, even to the point of experimentation. Again, this attitude was offensive to the traditionalists of the universities. All of these differences drove the natural philosophers, with their slowly developing ideas about the so-called *scientific method* away from the academics and toward the craftsmen of Europe. Thus, a blend began to form between the scientific method with its view of reality and the practical know-how of the Renaissance craftsman.

2. *Cooperation between classes.* The Renaissance has been called the age of adventurers and bastards. Many great men of the time, Leonardo da Vinci for one, were illegitimate. Most of these men were the issue of couples who had come from different social classes. In Renaissance Europe, classes were much more isolated than is so today and it has been suggested that Europe's artisan class had probably developed genetic characteristics which differed significantly from those of the nobility.

When individuals from two genetically distinguishable populations mate, their offspring is often superior in various ways to either of its parents, probably because the offspring carries a greater variety of genes. That the crossing of normally isolated Renaissance classes produced such a group of superior individuals is almost impossible to prove. Some geneticists feel, however, that this may have happened and that the mixing which took place so often in the Renaissance produced a large class of superior men who were in-

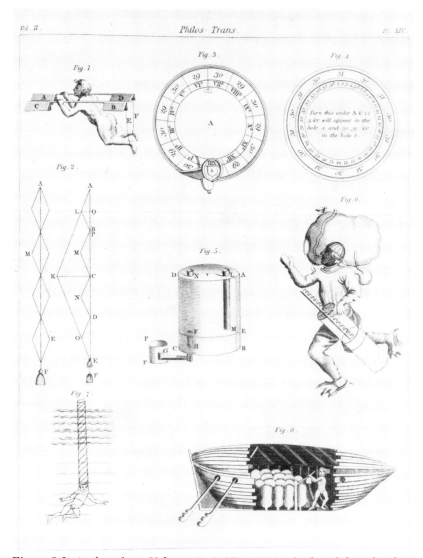

Figure 9-2. A plate from Volume II (1672–1683) of *The Philosophical Transactions of the Royal Society of London.* Plate shows: Fig. 1, a method of flying; Fig. 2, muscle structure; Figs. 3 and 4, an instrument for telling time; Fig. 5, a new kind of lamp (this contribution by Robert Boyle); Figs. 6, 7, and 8, methods for working under water.

strumental in forging science and craft technology into a working unit.

3. *The Renaissance economy.* A most powerful impetus for the union of science and technology came from the growing economy of Renaissance Europe. Expanding manufacture and trade, coupled with

the conquest of foreign lands, led to a demand for more accurate instrumentation and machinery. When joined with the existing technology, science proved an invaluable aid in achieving this goal. Early papers published by the Royal Society of London, a pioneer scientific group, provide documentary evidence to support this idea that science was joined with technology in an attempt to create better ways of doing things. From its very beginning in the seventeenth century, the Royal Society of London began to publish papers dealing with subjects such as ways of determining longitudes for navigational purposes, ways of refining ores, of pumping mine shafts dry, and of improving military weapons. Robert Merton, a sociologist of science, has found that less than half of the Royal Society's investigations concerned pure science; most were related to practical needs.

The practical needs of an expanding Europe thus helped to fuse the ideas and methods of pure science with the empirical know-how of technology.

In addition to the Renaissance itself, other factors have been suggested as instrumental to the rise of modern science-based technology. Two of these are the beliefs associated with the Puritans and the climate of Europe.

1. *English Puritanism.* Seventeenth-century English Puritanism looked with favor on science, for the Puritan ethic called on man to substitute passion with reason and appreciate God through the study of nature. Many of the early English scientists such as Newton, Hooke, Robert Boyle, and John Ray, the botanist, were Puritans. Of the sixty-eight founders of the Royal Society of London, forty-two were Puritans. Although we do not think of their work as such, much of what these men did was applied science—a union of science with technology. This was so because Puritanism looked with favor on all efforts to improve man's condition on earth. As a result of their beliefs, the English Puritan scientists thus formed a natural link between the ideas of science and the practical problems of technology.

2. *The climate of Europe.* The late Ellsworth Huntington, a geographer, linked the rise of modern technology to the climate of Europe. Essentially, Huntington felt that the climate of Europe (and North America) with its yearly and daily extremes has a kind of stimulating effect on its inhabitants that is lacking in other regions of the world. The Western European thus has been more of an achiever and has evolved a more sophisticated, science-based technology than is found elsewhere. There are some obvious arguments for this view. Perhaps the most telling argument against it is this: If Europe is in-

deed a superior climate for achievement of this sort, why did civilization first develop in the Eastern Mediterranean region and the Far East rather than in Europe?

CHARACTERISTICS OF MODERN TECHNOLOGY

In many ways a machine such as the stamping press shown in Figure 9-3 can stand as a symbol of modern technology and its characteristics. Here are some of these characteristics:

1. *Rationalism.* The stamping press was designed by technologists who combined their practical know-how with the more abstract methodology of science. Its operator may affix a good luck charm to the side of the machine, but other than this the press is assumed to operate on rational-scientific principles in a rational-scientific world.

2. *Power.* This machine, along with thousands of others, has given us a power base such as the world has never before seen (Figure 9-4).

3. *Complexity.* Not one in a thousand of those who read this book could run the machine shown in Figure 9-3. Of those who have run such a machine, not one in a hundred would be able to explain how all of its parts operate. Even the technologists who were involved in the machine's design would fail in this respect, for most would have

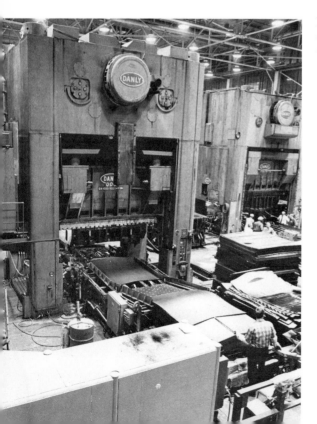

Figure 9-3. Press for stamping car hoods. (Courtesy of Oldsmobile.)

Figure 9-4. (On opposite page.) Energy available to technological man, as compared to that available to hunting-gathering and agricultural man.

Kilocalories in Thousands

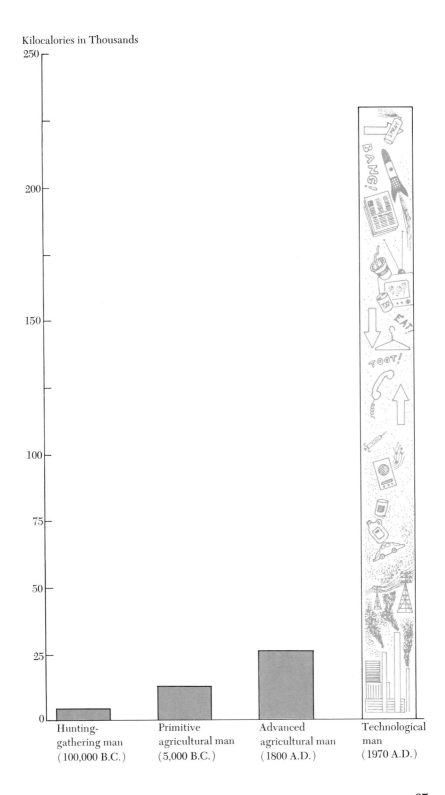

250

200

150

100

75

50

25

0

Hunting-
gathering man
(100,000 B.C.)

Primitive
agricultural man
(5,000 B.C.)

Advanced
agricultural man
(1800 A.D.)

Technological
man
(1970 A.D.)

been concerned with only one particular part of the machine. A Bushman understands his technology and most agriculturalists understand theirs. Our technology, however, has become far more complex. It is assembled and run by specialists, each of whom can understand or control only one aspect of the whole technological system. Generalists or holists are fast becoming extinct in our technological world.

4. *Impersonality.* The stamping press of Figure 9-3 has none of the personal qualities that a Bushman's knife has. The knife was made by, and belongs to, an individual. It can be recognized for its own idiosyncrasies of design. Its products, whether an arrow or a carving, are also personalized. In contrast, the machine stamps out the same product regardless of who pushes its buttons, and the products are all alike; they are anonymous. Anonymity is a key characteristic of the products created by our machine technology. If we look about us, the chances are that almost every object in the room in which we are sitting will be anonymous, for we have no idea who made it, where it was made, and we are often unsure of what these objects are even made of!

5. *Quantification.* The press of Figure 9-3 is a study in quantification. To mass-produce its products, that is, to create endless numbers of identical objects, it must be precisely designed. All its parts must be engineered to fit together and timed to work in union. Randomness is a dangerous quality to have in any truly successful machine.

6. *Change.* Almost certainly the press of Figure 9-3 is now, or soon will be, dated. One of the most striking characteristics of our technology is the rate at which it changes. Design improvements or changes in the wishes of consumers lead to never-ending modifications of all aspects of our technology.

7. *Isolation from nature.* Ultimately, the press is dependent upon the natural environment. It must draw upon energy to operate, and that energy is provided by a fossil fuel such as oil, gas, or coal. If one traced back far enough in time, doing a kind of family history of the press, its parts would all ultimately be traced to raw materials taken from nature. To the operator, however, this fact is unreal. The press and its near environment exist in a man-made world, almost completely walled off from the old natural environment in which man evolved.

Both our everyday lives and our everyday environment reflect the same qualities that are exemplified by the stamping press. Just as does the press, we exist in a rational world. We sometimes curse a chair after tripping over it. We may avoid walking under ladders or even

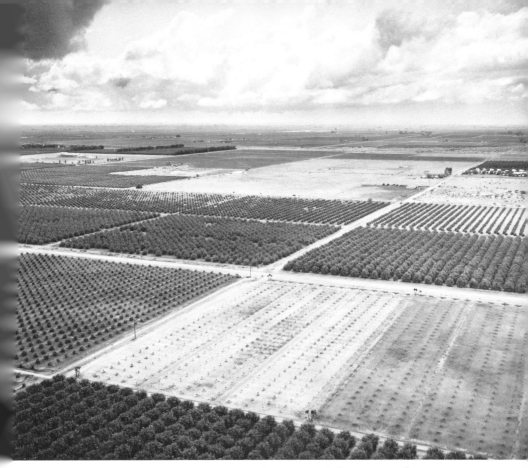

Figure 9-5. Citrus groves in Arizona. (Courtesy of the Bureau of Reclamation, USDI.)

talk about raging seas or angry clouds. But these are only leftovers from the animistic, supernatural world typical of the Bushmen and of our ancestors. Today we live in a world where all aspects of our environment, whether stamping machine, cloudburst, or riot, are to be explained in scientific terms. We have replaced animistic concepts such the Bushman's "people with no knees" with the impersonal, lawful concepts of science. The motion of the sun is now explained by gravity, inertia, momentum. No longer is the sun meat; it is an inanimate, impersonal body. The press stamps out metal not because it is angry, but because it obeys scientific laws.

Just as is true for the stamping press, our larger environment is characterized by power, complexity, impersonality, and quantification. With the tremendous power available to us we have reworked nature. Figure 9-5 depicts an American landscape from the air. It is interesting to compare it with the Bushman's environment (Figure 6-1). Our landscape is man-made; much of its flora and fauna is not native, and its topography is extensively remodeled from the original state. Straight lines are rare in nature, but the gridiron pattern, a precise, rectangular, measured, quantified, geometric arrangement of farm, road, and ditch, is a conspicuous feature of our landscape. Another striking feature is the sorting out which has taken place. Unlike the random mixture of tree, hill, and bush in the Kalahari desert of the Bushman, our landscape is typically organized into units—a field of alfalfa, a ribbon of concrete, a plot of grass. It is a mechanized landscape, reflecting the quantification, impersonality, and standardization that is so prominent a product of our powerful technology.

Quantification is also a conspicuous aspect of our daily lives; we think of it as time. The whole concept of time is an abstraction. Other than the approximate measures of seasons and lunar cycles, exact time is almost absent in nature. However, just as we have built quantification into our machines, we have also built it into our daily lives. We eat by the clock, sleep by the clock, and work by the clock. The clock itself is a machine, whose product is seconds, minutes, and hours.

Change is also a characteristic of our daily lives. Our fate has been to accept and even welcome change, which we have come to believe is synonymous with progress.

Finally, most of us are almost as isolated from the natural world as is the stamping press. We tend to feel that we are apart from and even above the natural environment. To Western man nature is an object to be utilized and transformed as he progresses toward his chosen goals.

What effect does our technology have on the natural environment and on the health of modern man? We explore these questions in the next six chapters.

10 MAN AND THE ENVIRONMENT: PROGRESS

THE NEBRASKA SOD HOUSE

My house is contructed of natural soil,
The walls are erected according to Hoyle,
The roof has no pitch, but is level and plain,
And I never get wet—till it happens to rain.
—from a Nebraska pioneer song

Sod houses were common on the plains of Nebraska and Kansas a hundred years ago. To build a sod house, a homesteader would first cut bricks of sod—Nebraska marble, as it was sometimes called—and lay them in tiers, grass-side down, to form the walls of his house. Doors were made of old planking and were attached with leather hinges. More often than not, the homesteader would use oiled paper instead of glass for his windows. The inside walls of a *soddy* were plastered, but the floor was dirt. The roof was always a problem. Planks were laid over a ridge pole of cedar, and a cover of sod was placed on the planks. Sometimes the weight of the roof collapsed the walls, or the sod slid off the planks. In any case, the roof almost always leaked.

Frontier life holds a certain nostalgia for most of us, but it was a hard, uncomfortable life. A typical sod house had the sparsest of furnishings. Bedsteads were built into a corner to save scarce wood.

CARL A. RUDISILL LIBRARY
LENOIR RHYNE COLLEGE

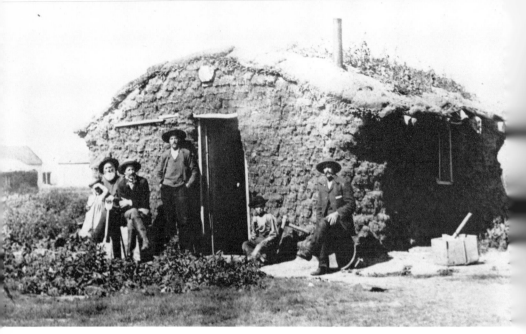

Figure 10-1. A sod house of the Kansas frontier. Note vegetation on roof. (Courtesy of the Kansas State Historical Society, Topeka.)

A table and a few chairs were thrown together using scrap lumber from packing cases. All sod houses had a stove of some kind for cooking and as protection from cold during the bitter winters. Usually the stove was iron, sometimes sod. Since wood was so difficult to obtain, the homesteaders used hay twists or *cow wood*, that is, cattle droppings, for fuel.

While the men worked their fields with hand-held plows drawn by teams of oxen, the women would do various household tasks, drawing water from the well, mending, cooking, and making soap. Clothing was of homespun or linsey, and hand dyed. Many homesteaders went barefoot in summer. If women went to a public meeting, they might carry their shoes and stockings until they were almost there, then sit down and put them on. In this way a pair of shoes could be made to last for years.

In one sense, food was healthful. As one Nebraska pioneer recalled,

I can't call up adjectives to describe the super quality of (corn) bread when eaten with "cow butter" or ham gravy, with a glass or two of rich milk or buttermilk made in the old wooden churn. It was simply "out of this world," as the youngsters today would say. So while we did not have frosted cakes, pies with two inches of meringue, and many other musts of today, we had food which met the needs of growing, healthy bodies and

102

we did not have to keep a bottle of vitamins from A to Z to keep us in good health.[16]

On the other hand, corn could get somewhat monotonous. It was a staple food on the frontier, a part of almost every meal. Wild greens and fruits were available in summer, but winter was a time of sameness, of salt pork, sorghum, and corn bread.

Family life was simple and, particularly during the long winter, monotonous. After the evening meal, the head of the family might have a pipe of tobacco or read from the family Bible, while his wife sewed or prepared food for the next day's meals. The children would do their chores and turn in early, for the morning's walk to school meant rising at dawn.

Vermin were everywhere. Bugs dropped from the roof into food, and biting insects, including fleas and bedbugs, were common. Even rattlesnakes sometimes turned up in a soddy's walls.

Although a few survive and are still in use, the prairie sod houses were largely gone by 1900.

Actually, the soddies represented a forgotten style of living that was reborn through the demands of the American frontier. Until relatively recently, the common man in Western society lived much as did the sod house pioneers. History tends to fool us in this respect, for due both to a lack of records and a lack of interest, our social histories have concentrated almost entirely on the life styles of upper- and middle-class people, ignoring the average man, who, after all, was in the majority. Until very recently, most of our ancestors worked with their hands for long hours, crafting their necessities from locally obtained materials. Their lives were harsh and often boring. In spite of his use of domestic plants and animals, the average Westerner's life was really not too different from that of a hunter-gatherer.

Things have changed a great deal in the last hundred years. We may complain about America today, but most of us would be loath to trade its excitement, variety, material wealth, and opportunity for a sod house existence. Our way of life, unprecedented in the history of man, is directly dependent upon the machine technology which underpins Western society. We will now look briefly at how this machine technology interacts with the natural environment.

THE AFFLUENT TECHNOLOGY

All material wealth is ultimately dependent on energy. With the unprecedented amounts of energy available through his technology,

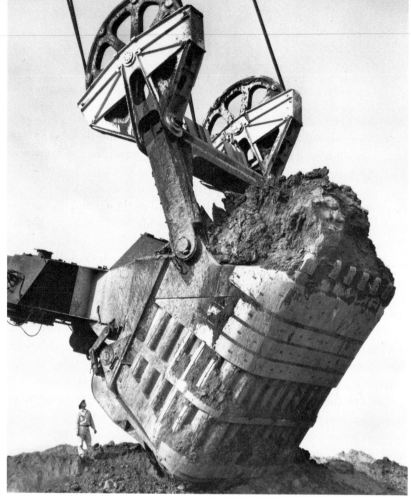

Figure 10-2. This dipper of a surface coal-mining shovel removes 210 tons of earth and rock a minute to expose underlying coal seams. (Photo by Bucyrus-Erie Company, courtesy of the National Coal Association.)

Western man has extracted raw materials and built them into machines to manufacture his goods and grow his crops.

About ninety-five per cent of the energy Americans use is derived from three *fossil fuels,* oil, gas, and coal. In each case, the fossil fuel is extracted and then taken elsewhere to be refined or utilized directly as a fuel. About five per cent of our energy comes from water power and nuclear reactors. Our consumption of fuel has multiplied thirtyfold since 1830 and hundreds of times since hunting-gathering days. Thirty years ago Buckminster Fuller estimated the amount of energy available to each American and decided that we each had the equivalent of 153 slaves working for us. Today, this figure is probably closer to 400.

Our country's demand for energy is doubling every fifteen years. America is by far the largest consumer of the world's energy. Every year we use almost two billion tons of oil, gas, and coal. Americans, who represent six per cent of the world's population, use about thirty per cent of the world's annual energy supply. About a fourth of this energy is used to power our transportation systems. Heating and industry are other major uses.

Much energy goes into machines which make things. Our sophisticated technology is now capable of producing a truly impressive range of goods. According to one estimate, the American economy uses over 2,500,000,000 tons of raw materials a year, almost thirteen tons per person. These raw materials end up as a continuously increasing cultural mass of cars, houses, electric shavers, shoes, and a thousand other items. The manufacture of all these objects creates a tremendous drain on natural resources. To cite one example, it takes 850 acres of

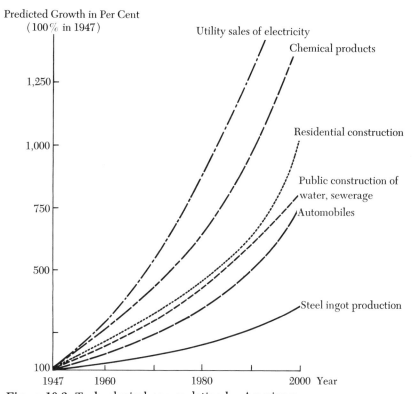

Figure 10-3. Technological accumulation by Americans.

Canadian timber to publish a single Sunday edition of *The New York Times*. (And incidentally, its costs the city of New York ten cents per copy to clean up the discards.)

A good part of the energy we use goes toward food production. While most of the world's inhabitants are undernourished, we have an overnutrition problem. Our bountiful harvests are directly dependent on the machine. With the aid of machines we have literally rebuilt ecosystems, rearranging their biota to suit our needs. Farms, cattle lots, and commercial orchards are examples of modern man-made *cultural ecosystems* specifically designed to produce food for man. We have also designed cultural ecosystems which supply us with non-edible products, such as wood pulp. To understand why all these cultural ecosystems have been so beneficial to man, it is necessary to contrast them with the structure of *natural ecosystems*.

WHY LAWNS?

Front lawns are an American institution. To most Americans, a house is somehow incomplete without its patch of green, modest though it may be. In some parts of the country, keeping a lawn requires prodigious effort. Flying over parts of the Great Plains, for example, one can see dozens of scattered farmhouses, isolated from each other by miles of wheat or corn. In front of each is a small patch of bright green, a lovingly tended, carefully watered oasis of grass, usually planted with a few trees and surrounded by shrubs.

Why do we do this? What does this highly artificial ecosystem and the work it demands provide that is worth so much?

One reason that comes to mind is children. Surely, a lawn is for play. This may have some truth to it, but how many of us have heard the words "Keep Off the Grass!" Perhaps then a lawn is really an object of prestige. This certainly has some truth to it, for that citizen who neglects his lawn is silently damned as a poor neighbor. Weeds and brown grass are a disgrace, and in some neighborhoods a kind of silent competition evolves in which each house tries to outdo the others in keeping its lawn trimmed, with its edges perfectly cut and every last offending weed removed.

In an interesting article, "Ghosts at the Door," John Jackson has argued still another function for the lawn. This function is beauty, but a particular kind of beauty. As Jackson sees it:

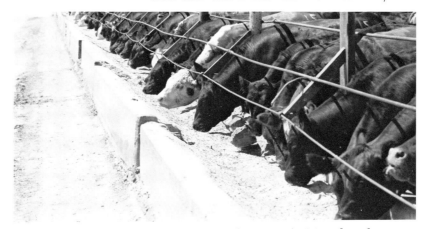

Figure 10-4. A cattle feed lot near Lubbock, Texas. (USDA photo by Fred S. Witte.)

"The front yard, then, is an attempt to reproduce next to the house a certain familiar or traditional setting. In essence the front yard is a landscape in miniature. It is not a garden; its value is by no means purely esthetic. It is an enclosed space which contains a garden among other things. The patch of grass and Chinese elms and privet stands for something far larger and richer and more beautiful. It is a much reduced version, as if seen through the wrong end of a pair of field glasses, of a spacious countryside of woods and hedgerows and meadow. Such was the countryside of our remoter forebears; such was the original, the proto-landscape which we continue to remember and cherish, even though for each generation the image becomes fainter and harder to recall." [17]

Jackson goes on to point out that our culture, at least until recently, was largely derived from northwestern Europe. For a thousand years after the collapse of the Roman Empire, the history of northwest Europe was one of slow and relentless landmaking, of wresting farm-land from the great forests which once covered the region. To Jackson, this was so basic a part of the European experience that we have carried a remembrance of the process and its resulting pasture and meadow into our present-day lives.

Perhaps the most striking difference between the two is the huge amount of machine energy which is involved in the maintenance of a cultural ecosystem. Farms and other agricultural enterprises use huge harvesters, combines, mechanical fruit shakers, irrigation sprinklers, pesticide-spraying helicopters, even road-building equipment to level fields for planting. Cattle feedlots utilize trucks to bring food to their stock and to remove waste. Helicopters pull lumber from commercial tree forests. In effect, all of these machines provide our cultural eco-systems with a source of energy much greater than that from photo-synthesis, which is the only form of energy available to a natural ecosystem. Not all of the energy we use to build and maintain our cultural ecosystems comes in the form of work energy provided by machines. The scientific and technological know-how which lies behind the ability to build and maintain a man-made cultural ecosystem also represents an indirect energy investment.

The two kinds of ecosystems also differ strikingly with respect to the species and food chains they contain. Natural ecosystems are typically complex in structure, with many species and many pathways for the flow of matter. In contrast, cultural ecosystems have been designed by man to eliminate all pathways and all species other than those of direct utility to him. Those species which he keeps in the ecosystem are often highly standardized to produce more efficiently for man's in-terest. Through genetic changes they have been designed to grow more rapidly or develop the proper size and shape. Many species have been tailored to fit the requirements of the machinery that tends or harvests them. Lemon trees are bred to grow to a prescribed height, wheat to ripen at a prescribed time. In California, ninety per cent of the tomato crop is picked mechanically. Huge harvesters cut and pull the plants, then shake off the fruit. To meet harvesting machine requirements, tomatoes are bred to ripen at one time, to have an easily snappable stem, and to have a skin tough enough to withstand bruising.

Genetic selection is often used to further man's specialized interests with respect to the kinds of products his ecosystems create. Some varieties of Southern pine tree, which supply most of our paper and pulp, have been bred to produce wood that is ideal for tissue paper. Other varieties produce wood for newsprint, and still others, wood for cardboard. Pine trees have even been bred to grow in a bent fashion so that their cones can be easily collected for seed purposes!

Western man has also redesigned the physical environment in which his captive species live. The cattle which are grown on feedlots (and eighty per cent of American cattle are raised this way) live in a

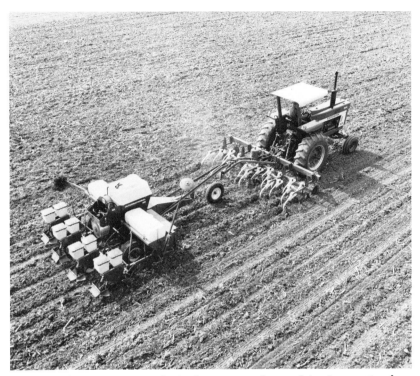

Figure 10-5. A four-row CYCLO planter manufactured by International Harvester. This machine is equipped with attachments for adding fertilizer, herbicides, and insecticides when seed is planted. (Courtesy of International Harvester Company.)

standardized environment. Food is carefully controlled for nutritive content and volume. The lots themselves are designed to avoid dampness and to have the proper temperature and exposure to wind. Easy access to feed mills and slaughterhouses is a prime consideration. The fields in most large American farms are highly standardized. Tailored to the demands of machine seeding, weeding, and harvesting, they have become larger and larger, their crop rows straighter and straighter (Figure 10-5).

In the most advanced cultural ecosystems both environment and crop have become almost completely isolated from nature. An egg factory is a good example of this. A typical egg factory consists of one or more buildings, often without windows, in which light, temperature, humidity, and ventilation are completely controlled. A large egg factory may contain over fifty thousand hens, arranged in rows of small

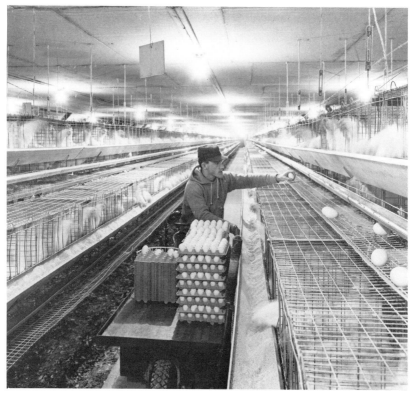

Figure 10-6. An egg factory. (USDA photo.)

cages (Figure 10-6). The hens have been genetically bred for maximum egg-laying efficiency. They thrive on food that is almost completely different from any their ancestors found in nature. For years, chicken nutrition has been an important field of scientific investigation, and the food used in an egg factory is a carefully measured blend of proteins, carbohydrates, vitamins, minerals, and medications to prevent those diseases which are a particular threat in the crowded conditions of the factory. Water and food are mechanically supplied, with feeding periods and volume of food regulated by a timeclock. Wastes are also removed by machine. After they are laid, eggs roll down a sloping floor to the collecting areas.

Sometimes a cultural ecosystem has some other purpose beside the production of food crops. A lawn is a good example. As most of us are only too aware, a lawn requires as much machine maintenance as any food crop.

Often Western man merely modifies, rather than completely redesigns, a natural ecosystem. For example, many farmers grow catfish or other edible fish in ponds. These ponds are managed by the addition of certain foods or the culling of unwanted fish in order to keep production as high as possible. While the pond ecosystem is thus reworked, it still retains much of the basic structure it developed through organic evolution. Other examples of human activities which result in the modification of natural ecosystems are oyster farming, the maintenance of maple sugar bushes, the creation and management of national parks, and the establishment of pasture lands.

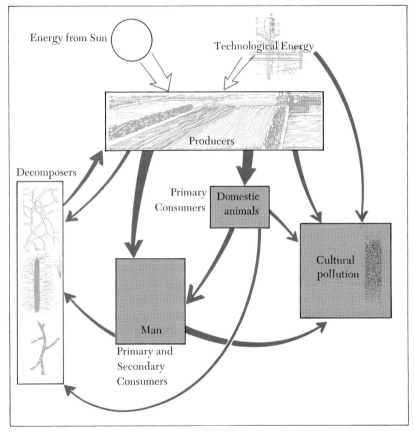

Figure 10-7. Flow of matter in a cultural ecosystem. Note that producer and consumer rectangles contain very few species compared to those of a natural ecosystem (Figure 1-6). The cycle characteristic of a natural ecosystem has been heavily modified, with much matter sidetracked into cultural objects, which act as pollutants, as will be described in Chapter 11.

In summary, then, Western man's technology has given him unprecedented power over nature. He has used this power to build a life of affluence such as no other men have ever enjoyed. While this technology is slowly spreading across the world, it is still largely confined to those Western nations which created it.

11
ENVIRONMENTAL PROBLEMS CREATED BY WESTERN TECHNOLOGY

Unfortunately, our material wealth and bountiful harvest have not been achieved without cost, for along with this affluence have appeared a series of ecological crises. Some of the latter, such as pollution and the destruction of natural environments, have been present as long as many of us can remember and are almost taken for granted as an inevitable part of modern life. Others, particularly the energy crisis, have appeared relatively recently.

None of these ecological problems are really new. To a varying extent, all have appeared in earlier periods of human evolution. What is unique to our era is the increasing scale of these crises and the fact that they seem to be converging into one generalized crisis situation.

Viewed in evolutionary terms, this crisis becomes understandable. For millions of years, representing ninety-nine per cent of his time on earth, man was a hunter-gatherer. During this period, he was in adaptive equilibrium with natural ecosystems, for hunting-gathering technology lacked the power to seriously disrupt them. Then, almost overnight, Western man developed a new machine-centered technology. This new technology has given him unprecedented power and has drastically changed his relationship with nature. His impact has had three consequences. First, since he has used his machine power to withdraw increasing amounts of material from nature, the natural environment about him is in danger of becoming depleted. Second, he has polluted ecosystems with the wastes of his affluence. Third, his alteration of natural ecosystems has not gone without dispute, for those plants and animals whose environment he has disrupted have proved capable of fighting back.

THE PROBLEM OF DEPLETION

Our capacity to capture increasing amounts of energy represents a kind of triumph, a new adaptive dimension which has given us the power literally to reshape the earth. From an evolutionary viewpoint, however, it is a most unnatural behavior. No other species has ever acted this way. The norm has always been a steady-state existence, a kind of partnership between species, with each using an unchanging amount of energy from generation to generation. Thus, our energy-growth curve is an aberrant and possibly short-lived event, a kind of lump in the usual flow of evolution. No other species has shown such a greed for energy, and there are increasing signs that our growth joyride is over.

Only a few years ago the term *brown-out* had not even been coined. Now these episodes of power shortage, with slowing air conditioners and dimming lights, are becoming a part of twentieth-century living, and worse may be in store. As this book is written, a national gasoline shortage has developed, and many experts in the energy field are saying that we are in for increasing trouble with respect to our energy supply. How long will the world's reserves of oil, natural gas, and coal last? At least three variables—the volume of yet-to-be-discovered reserves, the economics of using presently available sources, and changes in consuming habits—make predictions very difficult. Recently a House subcommittee made the following assessment of America's power situation: By 1985, demand for energy will be almost double that of 1970. Although coal still will be available, this increasing demand will result in massive shortages of natural gas and oil. This will be so even after a drastic increase in imports and development of new resources such as oil shales. Looking ahead still further, a prediction by M. King Hulbert of the U.S. Geological Survey sees ninety per cent of the world's gas and oil gone by 2035 and ninety per cent of its coal gone by 2300. Even if we were to discover some seemingly infinite source of energy, we eventually would run up against ultimate limiting factors in its use. For one thing, we can only build so many machines before we completely foul the landscape, to say nothing of the offence to our sense of aesthetics. Also, no energy source is completely efficient; all produce some waste heat. As we continue to build new energy production units, their waste heat will eventually alter our climate with disastrous results.

Food resources present as serious a problem as does energy; some would say a more serious one. Over the last twenty years, the gap between world population and food supply has widened steadily (Figure 11-1). Other resources do not present as serious a problem at this time, but they will ultimately do so if usage continues at the present rate.

Where does the greatest blame lie for the depletion crisis? Opinions differ, but the following factors have all been implicated.

1. *Increase in world population.* At the present time, the population of the world is approximately 3.7 billion. This figure has been increasing by about two per cent per year. Should current rates continue, the population of the world will double by the year 2006. In Latin America, Asia, and Africa, the rate of increase is well over two per cent per year. In North America it is 1.2 per cent, in Europe, 0.8 per cent. More people obviously mean increased use of natural

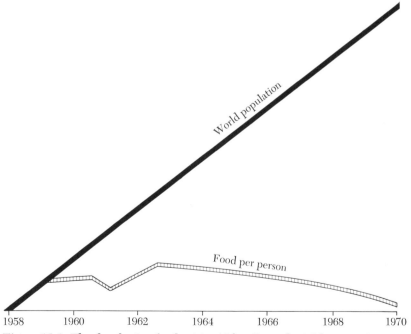

Figure 11-1. The developing food crisis. (After Benarde, Melvin A., *Race Against Famine*, Philadelphia: Macrae Smith Co., 1968.)

resources; thus the overall population growth of the world is an important factor in the depletion crisis.

2. *Resource use by the affluent countries.* The problem with (1) is that it does not take into account the fact that resource use is uneven throughout the world. Since the United States, with six per cent of the world's population, uses thirty per cent of the world's energy, we must bear more than an equal share of responsibility for the depletion crisis.

3. *The kind of goods produced by Western technology.* Since World War II, the production of synthetic fibers has risen by 5,980 per cent. The production of air conditioner compressor units is up 2,850 per cent, plastics are up 1,960 per cent, and electric housewares are up 1,040 per cent. In contrast to increases such as these, consumption of other items has fallen off. Among this latter group are lumber, down one per cent, cotton fiber, down seven per cent, and wool, down 42 per cent. The kinds of things in each list are highly significant, for they reveal a basic shift away from objects made with natural materials such as were typical of hunting-gathering technology to objects made with artificial materials. Most of the things our Western technology creates are artificial; a look about you will probably confirm this. Often it is impossible to identify the materials which go into the manufacture of the objects we use. This is even so for our food, for the chances are that you would have difficulty deciding what plants went into the manufacture of the breakfast cereal you ate this morning. Artificial objects have one characteristic in common: Their manufacture tends to draw more heavily on the world's resources, particularly its energy resources, than did the older natural materials.

4. *A way of life.* Basic values, ideas about what is important in life, are also involved in the depletion of natural resources. The American dream of progress has become diverted into a striving for more and more material things. This endless search for material wealth has produced our growth economy. It has also led to a throw-away economy in which material goods are continuously replaced by still newer and shinier things, which add still more to the drain on resources.

THE PROBLEM OF CULTURAL WASTES

As has been pointed out, nature has long produced its own wastes. The coal, oil, and other organic deposits we utilize for energy are really natural wastes, accumulations of material which have become

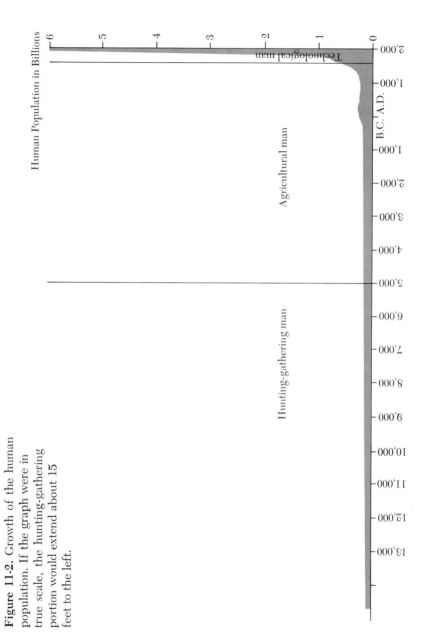

Figure 11-2. Growth of the human population. If the graph were in true scale, the hunting-gathering portion would extend about 15 feet to the left.

117

separated from ecosystem cycles. The bird droppings, or *guano*, found in deposits up to one hundred feet thick on islands off Peru provide another example of matter sidetracked from the normal recycling process of ecosystems.

Are these accumulations a form of natural pollution? After all, there is not that much difference between an accumulation of bird and human dung, and we would certainly think of the latter as pollution. It would seem that pollution is one of those terms which is much easier to use than to define. If we wish, we can define pollution as any waste which has accumulated through the action of living things. This definition, however, fails to differentiate between processes that are natural in the sense of having been present throughout all of organic evolution and those which have arisen through the action of culture. Since the latter are the source of our pollution problems today, we will use a somewhat more restricted definition and consider pollution to be any accumulated waste which is produced through the cultural activities of man.

As we have suggested earlier in the book, man has always polluted. Middens, or giant shell heaps along our coastlines, are nothing more than garbage dumps left by generations of Indian camps. The mounds found throughout the Near East which contain buried cities are literally built of garbage. Until very recently, however, man's pollutants were localized and could be absorbed by natural ecosystems. As cities became industrialized the pollution problem began to increase and in the last thirty years has reached explosive proportions.

All of our pollutants have one effect in common. In one way or another, they act to disrupt natural ecosystems. Pollutants can be classified according to the way they affect these systems. *Biocides* are chemicals which kill many kinds of organisms, thus causing an upset in the balance of species within an ecosystem. *Organic wastes* are materials which become incorporated into and upset the nutrient flow of an ecosystem. *Inert wastes* are materials which are not readily incorporated into ecosystem cycles. Western technology dumps great concentrations of inert wastes into natural ecosystems, literally smothering them.

Biocides

The chlorinated hydrocarbon DDT was first used during World War II. Millions of men, women, and children in the European war zone were dusted with DDT to rid them of the human body louse, which among other things carries typhus. The result was a dramatic decline in disease—for the first time in any major war more people were killed through combat-related causes than from disease. Since the war, millions of lives have been saved through the suppression by DDT of mosquitoes and other disease carriers.

Following its success against insect carriers of disease, the use of DDT was quickly extended to the control of plant pests of various kinds. At first, DDT and similar compounds seemed the long-sought answer to pest-control. But then some unanticipated problems appeared. Shortly after World War II, something began to happen to bird populations in the United States. A number of species, from the common robin to the bald eagle, decreased dramatically. All investigations of this decline pointed toward DDT as the major culprit. Studies

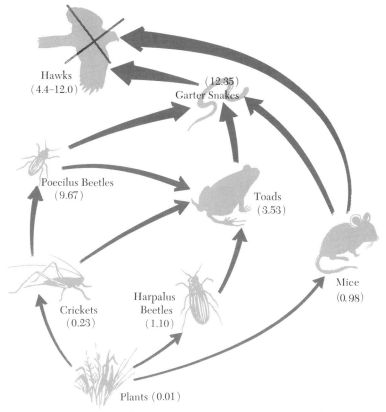

Hawks
(4.4–12.0)

(12.35)
Garter Snakes

Poecilus Beetles
(9.67)

Toads
(3.53)

Mice
(0.98)

Harpalus
Beetles
(1.10)

Crickets
(0.23)

Plants (0.01)

Figure 11-3. How a biocide concentrates in an ecosystem. Values are in parts per million. Arrows widen to suggest increasing concentrations which become lethal when biocide reaches hawks. (After Wurster, Charles F., "Aldrin and Dieldrin," *Environment*, 13, October 1971, pp. 33–45.)

showed that when DDT was sprayed on trees to control Dutch Elm disease, much of the spray fell on the soil beneath the trees. The DDT in this residual spray was picked up by earthworms and other soil-dwellers and passed via the food chain to birds. At each step the concentration of DDT increased. In many cases this concentration was great enough by the time it reached the birds to be lethal. Some birds, such as falcons and eagles, could tolerate the DDT in their tissues but produced eggs with abnormally thin shells, which often broke prematurely. In either case, the populations of affected birds declined drastically. The behavior of DDT in ecosystems has been studied intensively and is relatively well known. Its action seems typical of a wide range of biocides which man has introduced into natural ecosystems or into his own environment. Some of these, such as DDT, aldrin, lindane, and dieldrin, have been deliberately introduced to control pests. Others, such as mercury or lead compounds or even radioactive materials, have been inadvertently introduced as industrial or household wastes. In all cases, the biocide tends to pass from organism to organism in the food chain of an ecosystem, becoming increasingly concentrated until its effects are lethal.

Whatever pathway a biocide takes, its ultimate effect is to disrupt the checks and balances found in most natural ecosystems. Wagner cites a case in which Montana spruce trees were sprayed to control the Englemann spruce beetle. Red spider mites, which live in web-like structures on the underside of the spruce needles, were protected from the spray, but another mite, an enemy of the spider mite, was killed off. The following year the spruce trees were free of the Englemann spruce beetle but were heavily damaged by a huge population of red mites which were no longer held in check by their enemy.

Where does a biocide finally come to rest? At least in the case of DDT, large quantities seem eventually to leave ecosystem cycles and move to the atmosphere and ocean deeps. The implications of this concentration of DDT and possibly other biocides are not clear.

Organic Wastes

Before 1900, Lake Erie supported a thriving commercial fishery and produced millions of pounds of sturgeon, whitefish, herring, pike, and other species annually. But around 1900 something began to happen to Erie's ecology. The first signs of trouble appeared in the form of greatly reduced catches. The sturgeon catch, for example, dropped from a million pounds annually to less than 100,000 pounds a year by 1910. The same thing happened to other lake fish. Herring fell from

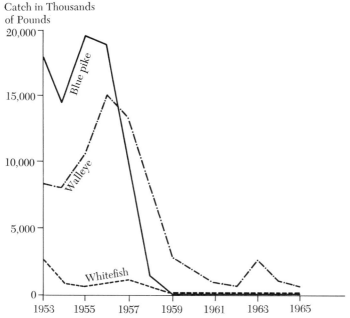

Figure 11-4. Decline in the numbers of commercially valuable fish in Lake Erie, 1953–1965. (After Powers, Charles F., and Andrew Robertson, "The Aging Great Lakes," *Scientific American,* 215, November 1966, pp. 95–100.)

49 million pounds in 1918 to one thousand pounds in 1965, whitefish from a high of seven million pounds in 1949 to six thousand pounds in 1965. New species, often of less commercial value, appeared to take the place of the older species. At the same time, other indications of trouble appeared. Great blooms of algae appeared in the summer to clog the lake, especially in its western reaches. Gunk of all kinds, including oil, human sewage, and dead animals accumulated along Erie's shoreline and a new ecosystem member, the scavenging rat, appeared. By 1967 a third of the south-shore beaches were declared health hazards and were closed to swimming.

What had happened to upset Lake Erie's ecology? Before the intervention of man, Lake Erie's ecosystem had existed in a balanced, steady state. Over some twelve thousand years an ecological cycle had developed, similar in form to that of most freshwater lakes. A variety of producer plants, both rooted species and floating algae, supported primary consumers such as small crustaceans and other plankton. Secondary consumers, mostly fish, fed on these. Decomposers, mostly bacteria and fungi living in sediment on the floor of the lake, completed the cycle. These decomposers attacked the organic debris formed by the plants and animals of the lake, reducing it to inorganic compounds. These then were reutilized by the algae to continue the cycle.

In order for the cycle to operate successfully, a large amount of oxygen was needed to support the plants and animals in the food chain. Thus, a delicate balance existed between the number of lake organisms and the amount of available oxygen. The decomposers were in a particularly precarious position, for during the summer Lake Erie tends to become stratified, that is, water circulation between the surface and lower lake waters largely ceases. When this happens, there is no way for additional oxygen to be pulled into the deeper regions of the lake, and the organisms residing there must rely on the oxygen already present. Over thousands of years deep-water organisms had become adapted to this limitation, and their numbers were matched to the amount of oxygen available to support them through the summer. The advent of urbanization, industrialization, and intensive farming along Lake Erie's shores has upset the delicate balance between oxygen and organisms. Twenty-five million people along Lake Erie now pour all sorts of organic material into the lake. Cities contribute millions of gallons of sewage and garbage every day. Farms and lawns contribute fertilizers, and other major contributions come from industry.

How has sewage upset the lake's balanced ecosystem? This organic matter is waste to us, but it represents food to the lake's algae. Our organic wastes are rich in nutrient matter, especially nitrogen and phosphorous compounds. In effect we are fertilizing the lake's algal population. As a consequence, a population explosion takes place, which we observe as an annual bloom of algae. This bloom turns Erie's shores green and depletes the upper waters of oxygen. These thick blooms of algae die off rather quickly and sink to the lake floor, where they disrupt the delicate balance existing there. The decomposer organisms on the lake's floor are overwhelmed by the massive amounts of accumulating algal matter. In their efforts to reduce the dead algae to inorganic chemicals the decomposers exhaust the oxygen in the lake's lower levels. As a result, the fish and other organisms which are adapted to life in the lower parts of the lake die from a lack of oxygen, contributing further to the accumulating layers of lake-floor debris. Over the years many feet of organic sludge has accumulated on the floor of Lake Erie. This organic debris has been bound into an inactive state by ferric iron. Some ecologists think that low oxygen levels tend to disrupt this inactive state, which poses the danger of large amounts of bottom sludge becoming free to pollute Lake Erie further. Actually, our pollutants are familiar substances to a natural ecosystem, for Lake Erie is adapted to process the kind of material present in our organic wastes. In fact, it must have them as nutrients if its biota is to survive. The problem results not from the kind of matter introduced, but from its volume. Naturally evolved ecosystems simply are not adapted to process the volume of organic waste which our culture produces.

In most undisturbed lakes, a slow enrichment or *eutrophication* takes place as more and more sediment gradually accumulates on the lake bottom. Eventually a lake becomes filled with sediment and ceases to exist. What has happened to Lake Erie is a drastic acceleration of this normally slow process, a cultural eutrophication which has taken place so rapidly that the lake's organisms have had no time to adapt themselves to the changes involved. The result has been a disruption and breakdown of Lake Erie's ecosystem.

At least a third of the 100,000 lakes in the United States show signs of cultural eutrophication, and a similar upset of ecosystem cycles can be assumed to be taking place in many terrestrial ecosystems which receive excess organic wastes from our cultural activities.

Inert Wastes

Every year American towns and cities collect 200 million tons of trash from their citizens. Americans dispose of seven million cars, 26 billion bottles, 48 billion cans, 20 million tons of paper, and 25 million pounds of toothpaste tubes. In 1969 an average American family used and then discarded a ton of empty packages. Commercial establishments were also busy accumulating trash. In one year the Colonel Sanders Kentucky Fried Chicken chain dispensed over 20 million plastic containers, 30 million paper-board buckets, and 110 million paper dinner boxes.

The volume of our waste is rapidly increasing. Part of this increase stems from the increasing number of goods we produce, but it is also due to the fact that we are becoming a throw-away society. All sorts of objects, from cars to razor blades, are designed to be used only for a limited time and then discarded. At one time a pen, if cared for, could be used for a lifetime. When ball point pens first were introduced they were designed to utilize a replaceable ink filler. Now the whole pen is discarded when the ink is gone. We can buy paper dresses,

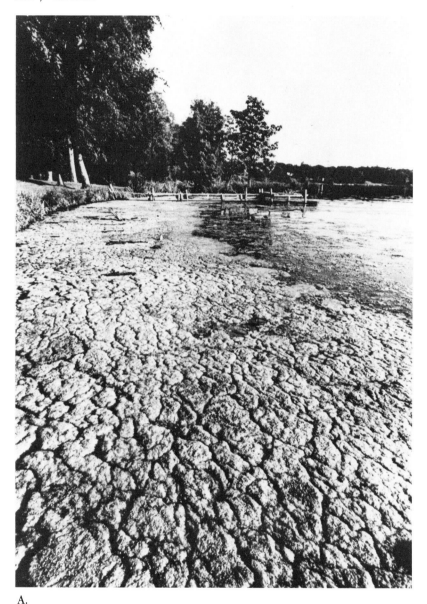

A.

Figure 11-5. A. Eutrophication of Lake Minnetonka in Minnesota, with layers of dead and dying algae along the shore line, prohibiting any life in these waters. The algae feed off nutrients poured into the lake from cesspools and sewage treatment plants. (Courtesy of E.P.A.-Documerica and *The Minneapolis Star*.) B. Eutrophication in Lake Tahoe, at California-Nevada border. (Courtesy of E.P.A.-Documerica/Belinda Rain.) C. Another result of eutrophication—dead fish by the thousands in a polluted stream in Illinois. (Courtesy of E.P.A.-Documerica.)

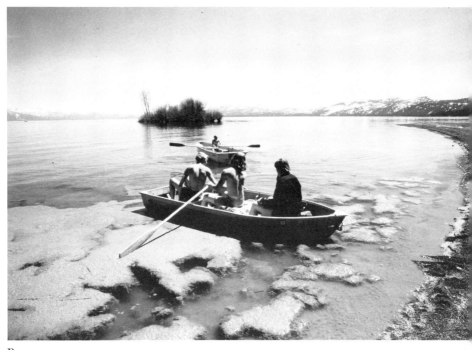

B.

C.

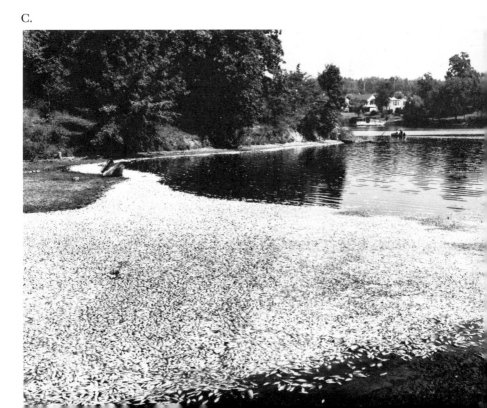

paper jewelry, even paper diapers, all to be discarded. The most publicized example of our throw-away economy is of course the non-returnable bottle.

A good bit of the waste we produce is still of the organic variety, but more and more Western technology is producing a new sort of waste composed of inert materials such as treated paper, plastics, aluminum, glass, and concrete. Discarded objects which are built of these materials are essentially inert, at least as far as an ecosystem is concerned. What effect do these wastes have? Since this new kind of waste is not readily incorporated into an ecosystem cycle, a junkpile of this material has a kind of smothering effect. Since ecosystems have great regenerative powers, new ecosystems eventually will develop around an accumulation of inert waste. Plants will force their way into the mass; animals use it for nesting sites. In a sense, then, man's inert wastes act as a physical environment for the ecosystem. The problem posed by inert wastes is that they are growing so rapidly that this regenerative process simply cannot keep up.

What eventually happens to all this inert waste? Much simply accumulates. For example, oceanographers in an isolated part of the Pacific recently recorded seeing 53 man-made floating objects over an eight-hour period. More than half were plastic. They estimated that between 5 and 35 million plastic bottles are now afloat in the Pacific. With time, however, much of this material probably is broken up by physical or chemical action and becomes dispersed throughout the physical environment. Beach sands, for example, have been found to contain small multicolored grains which are not sand at all, but microscopic bits of plastic. A study of offshore water from Maine to Georgia revealed microscopic fibers, apparently the residue of toilet paper.

Mixed Pollutants

Often, man-made pollutants do not fit neatly into one of the three categories we have described, but have characteristics of more than one of these. Crude oil spills are a good example. While oil is an organic material and is even a part of some ecosystems, its presence in large quantities has the same smothering effect as do our inert wastes. Oil spills, incidentally, are not new. There are reports of spills from sailing ships which carried crude oil, and during World War II, ships carrying millions of tons of oil were sunk. However, just as with man's other pollutants, oil spills are on the increase. One estimate is that 7,500 spills now occur annually, and when the anthropologist

Thor Heyerdahl crossed the Atlantic in 1970 on the Ra, he often saw oil slicks in midocean.

Polluting the Biosphere

The earth is in effect one huge ecosystem, the biosphere. Because of this, many pollutants are not confined to the area where they were produced but are transferred from ecosystem to ecosystem and thus are widely spread over the earth's surface. Some of these pollutants are disseminated by transfer along ecosystem pathways, but most of them travel via water or air. A pollutant will often follow unexpected pathways as it moves from ecosystem to ecosystem. Barry Commoner in his book *Science and Survival* cites a classic example of this. When nuclear tests were carried out in the 1950's it was assumed that radioactivity from fallout would concentrate around the test areas but be light elsewhere. After tests in the western United States, Eskimos in the far Arctic turned up with entirely unexpected concentrations of radioactivity in their tissues. As had been predicted, the Arctic soil was found to be much lower in radioactivity than the ground around the test sites. An examination of the Arctic vegetation, however, produced an unforeseen finding. Lichens, the predominant plants of the region, had a heavy concentration of radioactivity. Subsequent tests showed lichens to differ from most vegetation in their ability to capture fallout directly from the air, thus accounting for their high radioactivity. Arctic caribou live on lichens, while Eskimos eat considerable amounts of caribou meat. Thus, an unanticipated sequence of events led to dangerous concentrations of a biocide thousands of miles from its origin.

Our technology produces a complex variety of pollutants which enter the atmosphere. Homes, industry, and vehicles (including jets) collectively produce hundreds of millions of tons of pollution in the form of smoke, dust, and chemical droplets, particularly the oxides of sulphur, carbon, and nitrogen. What effect does this atmospheric pollution have on the world's biosphere? Some air pollutants consist of lead compounds. These can combine with iodine, a natural constituent of the atmosphere, to form lead iodide. When seeded into a super-cooled cloud, lead iodide crystals form nuclei for the condensation of rain droplets or snowflakes. Some meteorologists think that through lead pollution we are inadvertently seeding the world's atmosphere on a global scale, thus increasing the world's precipitation level. Jet contrails, those patterns of progress in the sky, may be another dangerous atmospheric pollutant. Under the right conditions, contrails do not disappear but instead form cirrus clouds. It has been suggested that several hundred supersonic jets would produce a cirrus cloud cover along their routes, with unpredictable results on the world's weather.

Dust may also have an effect on the world's climate. This is suggested by evidence from La Porte, Indiana, a town thirty miles east of Gary and South Chicago. The latter are steel (and thus pollution) centers of the Midwest. Since 1925, but particularly since 1965, La Porte has had a thirty to forty per cent increase in precipitation, a change which is very possibly due to the dust and other atmospheric pollution produced by its upwind neighbors. This supposition is strengthened by the fact that bad weather at La Porte correlates with days when pollution is particularly bad in the steel cities to the west.

Carbon dioxide, which is a major component of atmospheric pollution, may also be helping to alter the world's climate. Although the amount of carbon dioxide in our atmosphere has apparently varied greatly during the earth's evolution, these changes have been very slow, and the earth's ecosystems have had time to adapt. The potentially disruptive effect of carbon dioxide thus rests not on its volume, but on its rapid appearance.

In the last century man's fuels have contributed over 350 billion tons of carbon dioxide to the world's atmosphere, and it is estimated that we will dump a trillion tons by 2000 A.D. This rapid increase in

SYNERGISTIC EFFECTS

Dealing with the environmental crisis would be much easier if we could predict the impact of a certain action before it takes place. Unfortunately, ecosystems, and the plants and animals which constitute them, are so complex that our pollutants often have entirely unexpected effects. The unanticipated pathways taken by DDT, the ecosystem upset after spruce trees were sprayed, and the wanderings of fallout are some examples cited in this chapter.

Another sort of unanticipated environmental problem which is often encountered is the *synergistic reaction*. A synergistic reaction is one in which two or more separate insults to the environment interact to produce problems beyond those each will create alone.

carbon dioxide pollution may accelerate the so-called *greenhouse effect*. Just as does the glass of a greenhouse, atmospheric carbon dioxide reflects back those heat waves which are radiated by the earth's surface. The greater the concentration of carbon dioxide, the greater is this holding power and the greater will be the earth's surface temperature. Ecologists have noted that should the earth's average temperature rise by a mere 4°C., the polar icecaps would begin to melt and ocean levels would rise by over 400 feet, swamping many major cities of the world.

To many climatologists, the real danger from pollution will not come from the greenhouse effect, but from the dust associated with atmospheric pollution. This dust increases the world's cloud cover, and this may act to lower its temperature. At the present time we simply do not know enough to say just what long-range effects our changes of the earth's atmosphere will have, but we do know enough (or at least we should) to suspect that whatever they may be, they will probably cause problems.

ECOSYSTEMS FIGHT BACK

Not all natural ecosystems are complex and stable. Fire, wind, or flooding can destroy a natural ecosystem. When this happens, the affected ecosystem will pass through a series of evolutionary or *successional* stages. Immature ecosystems are formed first. These re-

An example of synergy may be helpful. When metallic mercury is dumped into lakes, it causes relatively little harm. However, if organic pollutants are also dumped into the same lake, the mercury will become a problem. The organic pollutants greatly increase the numbers of bacteria on the lake bottom. When concentrated enough, the bacteria begin to convert the metallic mercury into methyl mercury, which can be absorbed by fish and other lake dwellers, thus creating a new hazard to the lake's ecosystem. It is worth noting that as both our numbers and the complexity of our technology increase, the chances for cultural pollutants to interact, and thus the chances for synergistic reactions to take place, will also increase.

semble our cultural ecosystems is being unstable and simple in structure. These immature ecosystems will gradually evolve into mature ones, characterized by complexity and stability. Mature ecosystems are relatively resistant to invasion by outsiders, since all *niches*, that is, places for making a living within the system, have already been exploited by some kind of plant or animal. In contrast, immature ecosystems, with their simple and unstable structure, are vulnerable to invasion by many species. Since a cultural ecosystem is held in a continuous state of immaturity by man, the result is a never-ending battle between those who guard our ecosystems and a horde of pests which seek to invade them. A stand of pure corn, for example, is a potential utopia for corn borers and other species which can exploit the corn plants for food and shelter. As many Americans know only too well, a lawn must be continually sanitized to protect it from plant or animal pests who would reorganize it if given a chance, bringing it back

INQUILINES AND PESTS

The gypsy moth was first brought to America in 1869 by a professor who hoped to cross it with a local silk-spinning moth to create a silk industry. Unfortunately, the gypsy moth escaped into the countryside and spread through an increasing part of the continent, so that now it is found in a large part of the eastern United States, causing damage to oaks and other trees. The main areas of damage have been in the cultural ecosystems, or *urban forests,* typical of our suburban areas. The gypsy moth is only one example of a great horde of plant and animal life which has crossed the oceans to occupy our modified ecosystems. Some of these have been here for generations and are old Americans. Others, such as the fire ant of the Southeast, are new arrivals. Still others, such as the giant African snail, gained temporary footholds in the United States but subsequently have been repulsed.

The list of successful invaders is not limited to those which have colonized modified ecosystems such as our urban forests. Many species have colonized the more intimate environments of man. These—sometimes termed the *inquilines* of man—include a mixed bag of species such as the cockroach, silverfish, termite, housefly, black rat, and flour beetle. Some, such as the housefly, are often partial or temporary residents with man. Others, such as the German cockroach, have be-toward a stable situation of variety and complexity. Sometimes this happens—a vacant lot is an abandoned cultural ecosystem on its way back to a natural state of stable complexity.

How serious is the threat from pests that attack man's cultural ecosystems? In extreme cases, an ecosystem can be almost completely disrupted by these pests. A classic example of this was seen in the swarms of locusts which plagued farms on the American plains during the last century. The Irish potato famine of the 1840's provides another example of what pests can do. During the years preceding the famine, increasing numbers of Irish peasants had been deprived of their ancestral land and forced to exist on what they could grow on the tiny plots they still retained. Irish potatoes proved to be one of the most efficient food crops for these people to grow, and many families came to exist almost entirely on the yield from their potato patches. Unfortunately, as is true of any monoculture, the potato patches were

come completely adapted to man's environment and must remain associated with him to survive. In all of these species, earlier behavior patterns and even physical characteristics have been modified to help the species adapt to man-made environments. Some inquilines, such as grain beetles or clothes moths, are highly destructive. Many have been implicated as *vectors*, or carriers of disease. On the other hand, some are essentially harmless.

These inquilines and pests have used a variety of means to colonize America. Airplanes often provide an ideal mode of transport due to their speed. In spite of quarantine measures, many potential pests arrive concealed within exotic plants or other imports. For example, potentially harmful wood-boring insects have smuggled themselves into this country in handcrafted articles such as wooden buttons. This process of using man as an agent of transport has probably been going on for a long time. Lindroth, for example, has demonstrated that a group of flightless insects probably reached the New World in ballast carried by sailing ships. These ships loaded rock ballast (and the insects) in Great Britain, then sailed to Newfoundland, where the ballast (and the insects) was dumped and replaced by salted codfish, which was taken back to Europe.

subject to pests. One was a fungus, the potato blight, which can multiply rapidly and destroy potatoes when unusually rainy conditions exist. When this happened in the 1840's, many potato crops were destroyed and over a million Irishmen starved to death.

Much planting in our urban areas consists of one or only a few species of trees; now we are seeing the consequences of this practice, as town after town loses its artificial elm forest through the fungus infection called Dutch Elm disease.

Even when pests take only a part of an ecosystem, the losses are staggering. According to conservative estimates, a tenth of the world's annual food crop is lost through the action of pests.

Western technology has developed a variety of defenses against pests, the most spectacular of which have been DDT and other organic pesticides. However, in developing these, we have failed to foresee two things. The first is the tendency for pesticides to disrupt an ecosystem, as was previously described in the section on biocides. The second is the power of natural selection.

Whenever a pesticide is used, a few of the target organisms are likely to carry mutant genes which provide them with some degree of resistance. Prior to the application of the pesticide, these mutations are of no use to their carriers and may even be detrimental. Once pesticides are used, however, these few lucky organisms are much more likely to survive than their peers and will pass more of their genes for resistance along to succeeding generations. When the organism involved has a short life cycle, resistance can build very quickly.

Strains of cotton boll weevil, tobacco budworms, and other crop pests have become insecticide resistant; the same thing has happened with larger pests. Rats are pests both of urban areas and of farms, and until now they have been successfully controlled throughout the world by a poison called Warfarin. Recently, however, a colony of poison-resistant rats was found living on a farm in New York. A concentrated effort is presently underway to exterminate the colony. As health officials have noted, experience with similar colonies which developed in England and Denmark has shown that, if unchecked, colonies such as these can increase six to eight miles in diameter each year. The standard way of combatting pest resistance has been to switch pesticides, trying to keep one step ahead of the pest.

We have treated various aspects of the ecological crisis as if they were separate events. As a closing point, we think it is important to emphasize that in reality the problems of depletion, pollution, and pest invasion are tightly interlocked, a common result of Western man's reworking of nature. Highways provide an example of this interlocking pattern. Highways are a form of wealth, one which we are rapidly accumulating. In building highways, we draw heavily on natural resources, and the sand used in concrete is becoming depleted in some regions. Highways pollute natural ecosystems, not only by smothering them, but by providing a pathway for vehicles which exude noxious gases. Finally, highway borders are in effect cultural ecosystems, composed of grass or ornamental shrubs and trees. Pests of many kinds continuously invade these ecosystems, and the highway spray crew is a familiar sight in spring and summer.

In summary then, Western man's technology has enabled him to accumulate great amounts of energy and wealth. Some of this wealth has been taken directly from nature; some is produced by the cultural ecosystems he has fashioned. Unfortunately, his activities have led to a generalized ecological crisis. His insatiable desire for more and more goods threatens to deplete the world's resources. His cultural ecosystems are unstable and must continually be protected from assault by nature. His wastes threaten to destroy the natural environment upon which he ultimately must depend.

12
TECHNOLOGICAL SOLUTIONS TO THE ENVIRONMENTAL CRISIS

Increasingly, the power and expertise of Western technology is being brought to bear on the problems of resource depletion, pollution, and pest invasion. In the following pages we will present some examples of technologies being developed or proposed to solve the ecological crisis.

RESOURCE DEPLETION

Energy

Of all resource problems, that of energy supply is most crucial. Unless we choose to evolve back into our ancestral place within natural ecosystems, with only the energy of photosynthesis to support us, we must somehow solve the growing energy crisis. Two major strategies can help us gain this goal.

1. *Using our present energy supply more efficiently.* American cars consumed 66 billion gallons of gasoline in 1970 and somewhere around twenty-five per cent of our total energy use went into them. A wide range of proposals is aimed at reducing this drain on our energy supplies. One ingenious idea, which has been studied by Lockheed Missile and Space Company, involves equipping cars with a flywheel.

A flywheel works on exactly the same principle as a gyroscope. Once set to spinning at a high rate of speed, a flywheel's inertial motion stores a great deal of energy which could then be tapped to help propel a car, thus reducing gas consumption.

Electric and steam vehicles have been reexamined and new fuel sources, such as hydrogen, explored. Increasingly, our need for large cars is being questioned. It seems probable that energy shortages ultimately will reduce the number of private vehicles; buses and trains use much less energy per passenger than does a car (Table 12-1). Furthermore, electric trains can be powered by energy which is generated at one location, a much more efficient arrangement than the use of cars, which must take their fuel supply with them. Those who have visited Europe know that rail travel there is comfortable and fast. By the 1980's, most of the crack passenger trains in Europe are expected to travel at cruising speeds of over eighty miles per hour. There is no logical reason why train service cannot be equally comfortable and fast in this country.

Most American housing has not been designed with energy conservation in mind. It has been estimated that improved insulation alone in commercial and residential structures would result in an energy saving equivalent to seven per cent of our total national energy use. Frost-free refrigerators use almost twice the energy of conventional units. Incandescent lights use three times as much electricity as does a fluorescent bulb. Lack of trees about a house can make it harder to keep cool, as can dark shingles instead of light ones. Life styles are an important influence—about a fourth of all new houses now are mobile homes. With their thin walls and limited insulation, they need more

Table 12-1. *Energy Expended by Various Forms of Transport*

Item	Btu° per passenger mile Urban	Intercity
Bicycle	200	
Walking	300	
Buses	3700	1600
Railroads		2900
Automobiles	8100	3400
Airplanes		8400

° British Thermal Units.
After Allen L. Hammond, "Conservation of Energy: The Potential for More Efficient Use," *Science*, 178, December 8, 1972, 1079–81.

fuel for heating in winter and cooling in summer than do more heavily built homes. Artificial construction materials such as synthetics or plastics require considerably more energy to produce than do natural materials such as wood. Sometimes this energy difference is surprising. Although a building with an aluminum skin may weigh less and be easier to maintain, the use of aluminum requires about five times more energy per pound than steel.

The waste heat produced in many industrial operations could be used to run turbines for the generation of additional electricity. This approach has been little explored because until now oil, gas, and coal have been cheap enough so that industry would rather use fuels in relatively inefficient ways than spend money to develop technologies that operate on the principle of reuse.

2. *Developing new sources of energy.* Conservation of energy through more efficient transport, industry, and housing is vitally important, but none the less is only a stop-gap measure. New energy sources which are in much greater supply than the traditional fuels and which inflict less damage on ecological systems must be found soon.

Methane gas is one energy source which has been suggested as a replacement for conventional heating fuels. One advantage of this gas is that it can be produced from organic wastes such as those created by the wine-making and canning industries. Feed lots, agricultural enterprises, even our houses, produce organic wastes which could yield methane. The most likely method would be to utilize microorganisms to ferment the wastes. Methane derived from waste is already being used on a limited basis. Some sewage plants, for example, utilize methane gas of this type to run their machinery.

Still another energy source open to potential exploitation is geothermal heat. Geothermal power plants tapping the earth's heat have been constructed in Italy, New Zealand, Japan, Mexico, Iceland, Russia, and California. Little exploration has been done, but a vast potential exists, particularly if other fuels become too expensive. Tidal energy is another power source now little exploited, but certainly open to further development.

Another idea, first proposed in 1920, has recently been revived. There are significant temperature differences between ocean surfaces and ocean depths. William Heronemus of the University of Massachusetts estimates that 7,500 energy-harnessing devices placed off the Florida coast could provide the United States with enough energy for several decades. In each device, warm ocean water would flow through a heat exchanger. There the heat would be removed from the water, causing a second fluid to boil, thus driving turbines and generating electricity.

It has even been suggested that we ought to go back to wind power. It has been argued that forty-five thousand windmills could provide adequate power for the New England states, but it might be that no one would wish to live there any more!

Nuclear power, of course, is another potential source of energy. Conventional nuclear power plants of the sort in operation today are fission systems—that is, they derive energy from the splitting of some heavy element fuel such as Uranium 235. Unfortunately, according to one estimate, an acute shortage of usable uranium ore will develop before 2000. One way around this problem may be to develop breeder reactors. These operate in a fashion that ensures that more nuclear fuel is produced than is consumed. Breeder reactors, however, generate still further problems, because of their rather complex struc-

BETTER LIVING THROUGH LESS TECHNOLOGY:

1. COMMUNES

How much energy do communes use compared to traditional family units? Some approximate figures were obtained by a study of twelve communes in the Minneapolis area.

Some striking differences were found respecting the kinds of appliances found in communes as compared to those of a traditional family. Although about one quarter of all Minneapolis households have air conditioning, none of the communes studied had this appliance. None of the communes had dishwashers. Only two had clothes dryers, which averaged out to 0.02 clothes dryers per person, since the twelve communes represented 116 people. The 0.02 figure is one eighth the national average. Many of the commune members probably used laundromats, but these, of course, use less energy per person than do private dryers, since they are in use all day.

There were 32 cars and 45 bicycles in the twelve communes. Gasoline consumption per commune member was about 36 per cent below the national average, and car mileage per individual was 68 per cent below the national average.

Over 80 per cent of American domestic energy consumption goes toward producing heat. This heat is used for cooking, hot water, and

ture. This characteristic makes them potentially more likely to undergo accident or malfunction.

Some technologists think that the most promising power source of the future will be a type of nuclear power that has yet to be developed. Nuclear fusion, the joining of two light atoms to produce a heavier one plus energy, has been accomplished in hydrogen bombs and to a very limited degree in the laboratory. There are formidable problems to be solved before this sort of power source will become feasible, but it seems only a matter of time. The advantages of fusion power are twofold: It takes only a small amount of fuel to create huge amounts of energy and the reaction is clean, releasing relatively little radioactivity. Nuclear reactors do release large amounts of heat, and no satisfactory solution to the resulting thermal pollution has been found. Nevertheless, it seems certain that more and more of our power will come from this source. Recently, much interest has centered on the possibility of using nuclear power to produce large amounts of

space heating. The communes depended primarily on gas heating and used 40 per cent less gas than traditional families, after corrections had been made to equate differences in dwelling size and number of occupants.

In accounting for the differences between commune and traditional family units, two factors seem to be involved. First, the commune members themselves were practitioners of a new life style with a strong ecological bent. Thus, a part of the commune efficiency would be a reflection of personal attitudes about waste and the need for material things. On the other hand, the commune members enjoyed approximately the same level of material-good possession as did a typical middle-class household. Thus, most of the economies were of scale—a large cooperating household can simply use energy more efficiently than the average two-and-a-half people of the typical Minneapolis dwelling unit.

Although only a tiny fraction of our population has adopted the commune way of life, it seems worth considering whether or not some of the energy economies typical of this life style might not be transferred to the single family.

hydrogen, thus creating a hydrogen economy to replace our predominantly electric economy. Under one plan, big nuclear reactors would be built offshore. These would produce electricity, which would be used to dissociate sea water into oxygen and hydrogen. The hydrogen then would be pumped ashore. Unlike electricity, hydrogen can be stored easily until needed. If it were burnt in pure oxygen to produce energy, the only pollutant would be water. We could thus free ourselves from smog, although we might create a humidity problem.

In many ways our best energy source would be that which supplies the power to drive all natural ecosystems—the sun. The use of solar power has long been a dream of man. A handful of scientists and technologists who have spent years on the problem say it could become a practical energy source. Dr. Erich Faber of the University of Florida's Solar Energy and Energy Conversion Laboratory has been developing all sorts of machines such as pumps, turbines, refrigerators, and house ovens powered by solar energy. In Florida some houses use water that is heated by solar-powered units. The units consist of a black-coated pan which is mounted on the roof. Solar heat is absorbed by water in the pan and then transmitted to water in pipes running through the pan. In this way enough hot water is produced

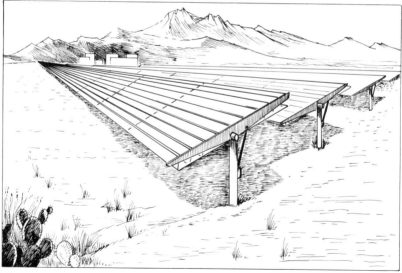

Figure 12-1. An artist's visualization of a solar power farm. (Courtesy of Optical Sciences Center, University of Arizona.)

to serve the needs of an average family. If used commercially, solar energy would probably be converted to electricity through the use of selenium or silicon cells. When sunlight strikes either material the solar heat is converted to electricity.

Another way to capture solar energy would be to develop land-based power stations. Drs. Aden and Marjorie Meinel of the Optical Sciences Center at the University of Arizona have suggested that a National Power Facility could be located in the Southwest. This facility could generate enough power to supply most of America's needs. Since solar energy would drive steam turbines, the latter would need fresh water for cooling. In the Meinels' scheme, ocean water would be brought in and desalinated for this purpose. Large land areas would be needed and some ecological problems might result, but the Meinels think they would be minor compared to the problems created by conventional power sources. In their plan the Meinels would use lenses to focus the sun's rays onto pipes coated with a heat-absorbent material. Nitrogen gas in the pipe would pick up this heat and pass it to a storage unit.

Other heat-capture systems also are being developed. For example, Ernst Eckert of the University of Minnesota and Rodger Schmidt of Minneapolis-Honeywell Inc. are working on a system which uses a parabolic reflector to concentrate sunlight. An even more imaginative system would be to place huge solar collectors in space. These would then beam electricity to earth via microwaves (Figure 12-2).

Whatever route we take toward solving our energy crisis, two points remain crucial: As of today, we do not have enough sources for our present and anticipated energy needs, and we have not as yet developed the technology necessary to tap new sources.

Other Resources

1. *Raw materials.* For the immediate future, raw materials such as iron, copper, limestone, timber, and the like do not seem to be as critical a problem as is energy. Ultimately, however, we will run out of these materials unless we radically rethink our technology. One goal might be to reduce needless obsolescence. Planned obsolescence makes sense in the case of some objects, such as a band aid, but cars or refrigerators do not have to be designed this way. Reducing needless obsolescence would help decrease our drain on raw materials and energy and would also help alleviate pollution. Another goal might be to redesign objects so that when we are through with them they can be easily reduced to basic raw materials and recycled. Developing

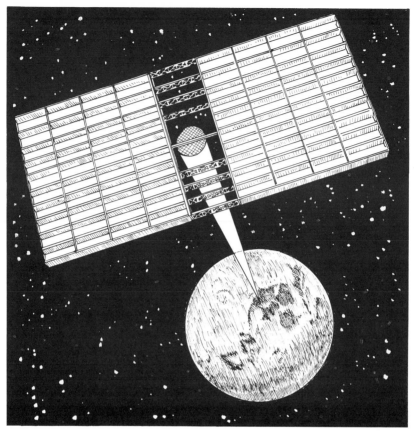

Figure 12-2. Artist's visualization of a solar power station located in space. (Courtesy of Arthur D. Little, Inc.)

ways of sorting out the components of our material objects is one of the most challenging problems of technological design. A tin can, for example, is composed of a layer of steel with a coat of tightly bound tin. A TV set is a tightly bound package of metal, plastics, and glass. Junked cars are even worse. Synthetic products such as floor tiles are often impossible mixtures which resist unscrambling. At present, the unmixing of such materials is too often uneconomical. Some day, however, the tremendous temperatures generated by fusion power could conceivably provide a fusion torch which could be used to re- duce these objects to their constituent atoms. These could then be reused, forming a cyclic closed technology (Figure 12-4). Even though the problem is formidable, technologies are slowly being developed to recycle our used materials. Some of these will be mentioned in the section on pollution.

Where are they now?

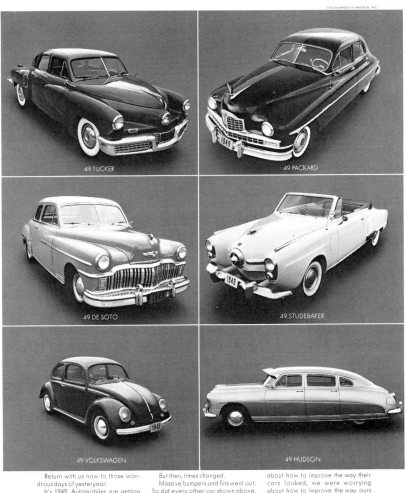

Return with us now to those won-drous days of yesteryear.

It's 1949. Automobiles are getting longer, lower and wilder.

Massive bumpers are a big hit. Fins are in. And everyone's promising to "keep in style with the times."

But then, times changed.

Massive bumpers and fins went out. So did every other car shown above, except the Volkswagen.

Why?

Well you see, back in '49, when all those other guys were worrying

about how to improve the way their cars looked, we were worrying about how to improve the way ours worked.

And you know what?

2,200 improvements later, we still worry about the same thing.

Figure 12-3. A Volkswagen ad of 1970. The obsessive American urge for newness helps increase the drain on natural resources. (Courtesy of Volkswagen of America, Inc.)

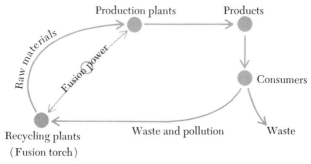

Figure 12-4. Fusion power could be used to create a "closed materials economy." Waste materials would be reduced to their constituent atoms, which then could be recombined into new products.

2. *Food.* While Americans and other westerners grow fatter, much of the non-Western world lives in a state of near famine. How serious is this crisis? Opinions range widely. At one extreme are pessimists such as the Paddocks with their book *Famine 1975!* At the other extreme are the optimists, such as those scientists of the United Nations Food and Agricultural Organization who have forecast that a hundred years from now the world can feed 36 billion people at our standard of living. Most food scientists fall somewhere between these extremes and see the world food crisis as very serious but not necessarily hopeless. The short-range goal of most is to buy time—to increase world food productivity to keep abreast of the growing world population, with the hope that the latter will level off before disaster strikes. How does one go about increasing food production? One tactic, much publicized under the term *Green Revolution,* is to introduce our agricultural technology into underdeveloped countries such as Pakistan, India, Indonesia, and the Philippines. Most emphasis has been given to increased use of fertilizers and development of new high-yield varieties of grain. The Philippines, for example, have been given new varieties of rice. The rice plant has been redesigned to make it absorb more fertilizer than the old native strains. It is also shorter in order to help it resist typhoon damage and to support the heavier head of grain which it produces. Rice fields have been redesigned to make them more efficient. Pesticides and harvesting machinery have also been introduced.

How successful has the Green Revolution been? Proponents feel it will buy enough time to stave off disaster, and there is no question that productivity has increased in certain of those countries where the new techniques have been introduced. Critics of the Green Revolution think it has given us a false sense of security. They feel the increase in food production has been achieved at a cost of the creation of too many new problems. Some new strains have a different taste than the old native strains and are not accepted readily. The new strains are not adapted to their environment in the way the old ones were. The old strains were hardy and would grow if left alone, while the new ones must be protected from pests, heavily fertilized, and well watered if they are to achieve their full potential. As a result, any deviation from ideal conditions—such as an unusually dry year—will drastically lower productivity.

The Green Revolution also brings with it the basic weakness of Western technological agriculture. The huge volume of wheat, corn, beef, and pork produced on American farms is not simply a result of superior technology. It is also dependent on the continual importation of raw materials. These imported resources take the form of fuels to run our agricultural machines, fertilizers for our crops, and even feed for our animals. Native agricultures use simple, locally produced implements, fertilizers, and feeds. In shifting to a Western-style agriculture, countries such as the Philippines, Indonesia, or India must also become dependent on outside resources. Thus, the basic problem the world must face is this: If we are to mechanize all of the world's agriculture, will there be enough natural resources to go around?

Finally, the Green Revolution implies a large-scale, sophisticated farming operation. This means that the wealthy landowner stands to gain more than the poorer peasant, who does not have the means to adopt the new kind of agriculture.

Other proposals for increasing agricultural productivity include clearing off forest land for crops and irrigating desert areas. These schemes might temporarily solve the food crisis, but many observers think that the world could not withstand the increased ecological problems they would create.

Population Size

We must develop new energy supplies, improve our ways of using raw materials, and grow more food. Yet none of these measures will have any meaning if we cannot control our own numbers.

1. *The technology of birth control.* Present-day birth-control technology includes the pill, the diaphragm, foams, condoms, IUDs, sterilization, and the rhythm method (if the latter can be called a

BETTER LIVING THROUGH LESS TECHNOLOGY:

2. MONOCULTURES

The insert shows an orchard-garden in the Indian village of Santa Lucia, Guatemala. Edgar Anderson, one of the leading botanists of our time, came upon the garden while he was in Guatemala studying corn. Here is what he has to say about this garden:

"The garden I charted was a small affair about the size of a small city lot in the United States. It was covered with a riotous growth so luxuriant and so apparently planless that any ordinary American or European visitor, accustomed to the puritanical primness of north European gardens, would have supposed (if he even chanced to realize that it was indeed a garden) that it must be a deserted one. Yet when I went through it carefully I could find no plants which were not useful to the owner in one way or another. There were no noxious weeds, the return per man-hour of effort was apparently high, and I came away feeling that as an experienced vegetable gardener (I am one of those strange people who would rather hoe vegetables than play golf or go to the movies) I had gotten more new ideas about growing vegetables than from visiting any other garden anywhere. . .

It is frequently said by Europeans and European Americans that time means nothing to an Indian. This garden seemed to me to be a

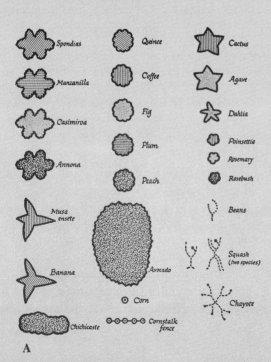

A. Symbols for a diagrammatic map of an orchard-garden in the Indian village of Santa Lucia, Guatemala. The ideograms not only identify the plants as shown in B, but they also indicate by their shapes in what general category the plants belong. Circular shapes indicate fruit trees (such as plum and peach) of European origin; rounded irregular shapes indicate fruit trees (such as the manzanilla) which are of American origin. Similarly, dotted lines are for climbing vegetables, small circles for subshrubs, and the irregular wedge-shaped figure for plants in the banana family.

good example of how the Indian, when we look more than superficially into his activities, is budgeting his time more efficiently than we do. The garden was in continuous production but was taking only a little effort at any one time: a few weeds pulled when one came down to pick the squashes, corn and bean plants dug in between the rows when the last of the climbing beans were picked, and a new crop of something else planted above them a few weeks later. . . .

. . . I suspect that if one were to make a careful time-study of such an Indian garden, one would find it more productive than ours in terms of pounds of vegetables and fruit per man-hour per square foot of ground. Far from saying that time means nothing to an Indian, I would suggest that it means so much more to him that he does not wish to waste it in profitless effort as we do." [18]

Anderson seems to imply that we would do well to investigate the possibility of developing an agriculture closer in its design to an Indian garden than to our present mechanized monocultural farms. If we had such an agriculture, could it adequately support our population, or would we have to greatly increase the number of farm workers?

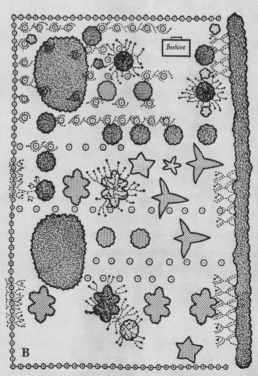

B. Map of the orchard garden. The long, irregular mass at the right-hand side of the garden represents a hedge of *chichicaste*, a shrub used by the Mayas. (Figures 13 and 14 from Edgar Anderson, *Plants, Man, and Life*. Berkeley: University of California Press, 1952. Reprinted by permission of the Regents of the University of California; originally published by the University of California Press.)

technology). New options are on the way. One of these may be an improved pill which would allow a woman to control the precise time of ovulation. A pill of this kind would have several advantages. It would probably be safer than the present pill, it would only be taken once a month, and it might be acceptable to the Roman Catholic Church.

Work is underway to develop a male contraceptive pill. Chemicals have been found which act to block sperm production, and these are being tested. Work is also underway to develop tiny valves which would fit into the male's sperm duct. These, if perfected, would make vasectomies reversible, eliminating one of the major objections to male sterilization.

2. *Using birth-control technology.* In the Western world, birth control is widely practiced and zero population growth now seems an attainable goal. In the United States, for example, the birth rate is now below replacement level. If it remains unchanged, our population should stabilize at 320 million by the year 2040. Less progress has been made in the non-Western world. The trouble is that people usually do not limit the number of children they have for altruistic reasons such as saving the environment. Instead, the size of their family is a function of their life style. In an urbanized mobile society such as ours, children become a hindrance to many couples. In non-Western agricultural societies children are valuable economic assets, helping on the farm and in the home. Life tends to be simple and family-centered. The old people of a community depend almost entirely on their children for support. In many agricultural societies a large family is a sign of virility and male sterilization is looked on with horror. All of these factors work together to produce large families. The question which haunts many population ecologists is whether the non-Western cultures can shift to the urban pattern in time.

If the non-Western world follows the pattern set by the West, it will not approach a state of population equilibrium until its material wealth has evolved to the level we enjoy. To do this, the non-West must greatly increase its use of natural resources, essentially developing a technology such as ours. Unfortunately, this may prove a difficult task, for in order to do this the non-Western world must compete with the West for scarce resources.

Suppose we are successful in halting population growth. What would an optimum world population be? According to one calculation, the world's ecosystems could support perhaps a billion people at the current American standard of living. Obviously an optimum population depends to a large degree on the life style or styles the world's inhabitants want. A recent symposium of scientists differed widely as to whether an optimum is even a logical concept. Perhaps the best viewpoint is that of Barry Commoner, who refuses even to consider the question, arguing that we have a much more important question to face: How can we slow population growth sufficiently to avoid catastrophe in the years ahead?

POLLUTION

Three basic strategies are available in the battle to reduce pollution of the environment by our cultural wastes. These are to recycle wastes rather than dumping them into ecosystems; to buffer wastes, that is, allow them to move gradually into ecosystems, and finally; to reclaim polluted ecosystems.

Recycling Wastes

In order to recycle wastes, they must first be collected. The sewage systems which transport so much of our domestic wastes are themselves wasteful. Not only do they require great amounts of water, but the liquid sewage which results is hard to work with. Various schemes have been or are being developed to replace water with some other vehicle. Every time we flush a toilet, we send a pint or so of human waste toward the sewer in five gallons of water. The Chrysler Corporation has developed an *Aqua Sans* system, which uses a special mineral oil rather than water for transporting human waste. The oil and waste is sent to a separator tank where urine and solids sink to a holding tank and are eventually burnt to a sterile ash. The oil is filtered, chlorinated, and returned to the toilet tank.

In Sweden, vacuum pipes are used to collect bagged garbage from apartments. The garbage is dropped into chutes in apartment-house walls and whisked to a refuse pile a half mile away, where an automatic process removes metal and glass. The remainder is burnt to provide heat for the apartments.

Attempts are being made to develop ways of recycling the organic wastes produced on farms and cattle lots. Most people don't think of cattle dung as particularly recyclable, but cattlemen wish it would be. A herd of twenty thousand cattle will produce eighty tons of waste a day. It is expensive to haul away, and since most farmers use chemical fertilizer, there would seem to be little market for cattle dung. John D. MacKenzie, an engineer at UCLA, has experimented

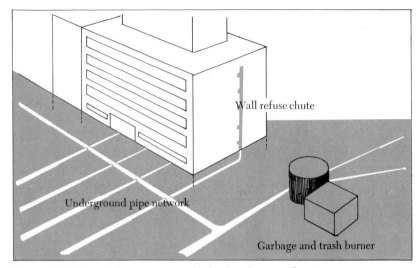

Figure 12-5. Swedish vacuum method of garbage collection.

with a mixture of treated dung and recycled glass which he heats and processes into bricks. These are odorless, can be sawed or painted, and are cheaper than ordinary building bricks. Another possible use for cattle or other animal wastes would be to convert them into livestock feed, and research is under way to make this an economical and safe process.

The recycling of bottles is one of the more publicized examples of an attempt to reuse inorganic waste. Instead of dumping used bottles by the roadside and so into an ecosystem, beverage companies ask their customers to return bottles to collecting points, thus keeping them out of nature and at the same time lowering the amount of new raw materials the companies need. However, recycling of bottles is not as straightforward as it might seem. For one thing, the public does not seem very eager to return used bottles. And in spite of the clamor, the trouble involved in recycling bottles negates the money saved. If bottles are recycled intact, they must be inspected for flaws, an expensive process, and must initially be made of thick glass. It has been estimated that bottles can make only about five round trips before they must be broken up. At present, about thirty per cent of all commercial glass is made up of *cullet,* or old crushed glass. In addition to use in bottles or other containers, cullet has been made into Glassphalt, a road surfacing material made of a mixture of asphalt and glass. It has even been suggested that old glass might be processed into artificial sand for beaches.

Since cars have become a part of the American landscape, 2½ billion used tires have been strewn about the countryside. The year 1973 alone added 240 million more. University of Wisconsin researchers have been developing a process to reuse these old tires. When frozen to —80°F., tires become brittle and can be powdered. The researchers suggest that twenty or thirty mobile freezer-crusher units might roam our countryside, collecting and recycling old tires.

Many other technologies are springing up to recycle organic and inorganic wastes; ultimately this would seem the most promising method of reducing pollution, particularly since it has the added benefit of reducing our draw-down on natural resources.

Buffering Wastes

Although we may ultimately build a man-made environment which recycles all its wastes, this would require much more technological

Figure 12-6. Aerators of a new design are used at the Quincy Industrial Treatment Plant in Quincy, Washington, to clean water. (Courtesy of the Bureau of Reclamation, USDI photo by J. D. Roderick.).

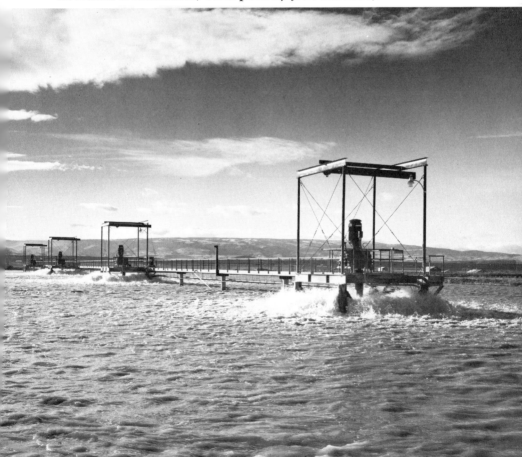

sophistication than we now possess. For the foreseeable future, we will continue to release a considerable portion of our wastes into natural ecosystems. Thus we badly need interim technologies which do not simply dump wastes into nature, but release them at a rate and scale which is slow enough so that the wastes can be absorbed without undue disruption to ecosystems. We are only beginning to explore ways and means of doing this. Probably one of the best examples of a developing technology of this kind, one which buffers or eases the re-entry shock of wastes, is to be found in a new kind of sewage system which is now appearing. Traditional sewage systems are designed to combat the foulness of sewage and its potential of spreading disease. Sewage is transformed into a mix of organic compounds that are neither dangerous nor offensive to man. Unfortunately, little attention is given to the fact that this processed sewage, which is in effect a fertilizer, is dangerous to natural ecosystems when released at a high volume into their pathways. The newer approach is to make the whole sewage system a kind of buffer which receives organic wastes

A.

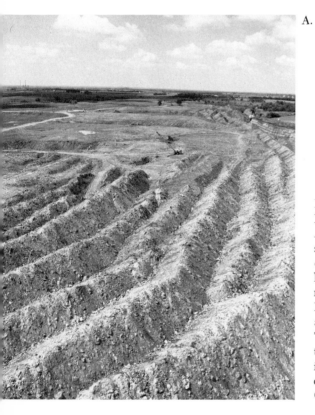

Figure 12-7. Strip mining in Henry County, Missouri.
A. Foreground shows newly strip-mined land, while top center shows mined land that has been graded and made ready for reclamation.
B, C. Strip-mined land adjacent to that shown in A. This area has been reclaimed to pasture and water impoundments. (Courtesy of the Peabody Coal Company.)

and passes them into either natural or cultural ecosystems at acceptable concentrations.

Reclaiming Polluted Areas

A third tactic in the battle against pollution is to develop technologies which reclaim polluted areas, turning them back to a reasonably natural state. Garbage dumps, for example, are often converted into various kinds of recreational areas. The reclaiming of land that has been strip mined for coal is another example of this approach. While we have no desire to defend strip mining, the growing fuel crisis may force us to use the coal reserves which are available through this kind of mining. If so, it would behoove us to learn as much as we can about ways to return stripped land to productivity. Experience in West Germany has shown that this can be done, and some progress along these lines has been made in the United States (Figure 12-7). Finally, there are encouraging signs that it may not be as difficult as it once was thought to be to return badly polluted

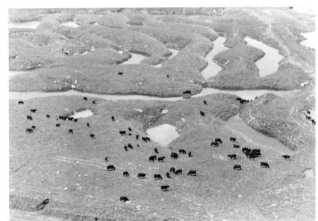

B.

C.

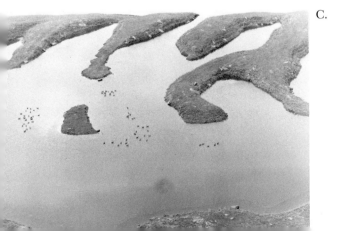

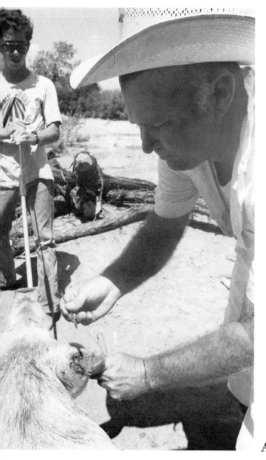

A.

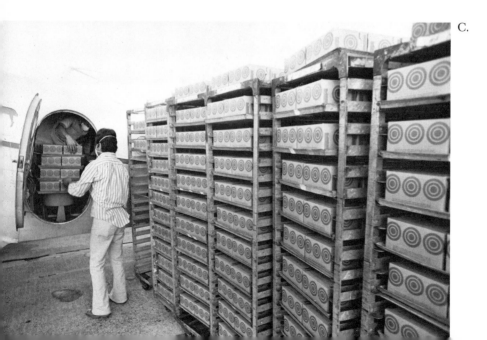

C.

Figure 12-8. Scenes from the U.S. Department of Agriculture Screwworm Eradication Program in Texas. A. Livestock inspector examines swine with infested wounds. B. Canister containing 18,000 fly pupae is placed in Cobalt-60 chamber for irradiation. C. Plane is loaded with cartons containing sterile flies. D. Dr. James E. Novy shows how box breaks open after leaving airplane, releasing 2,000 male flies. (USDA photos.)

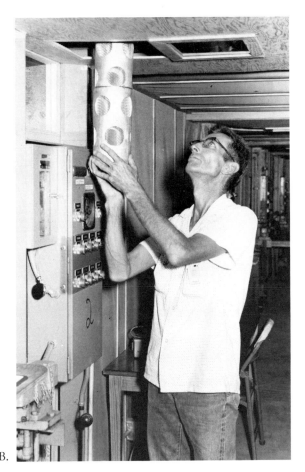

B.

D.

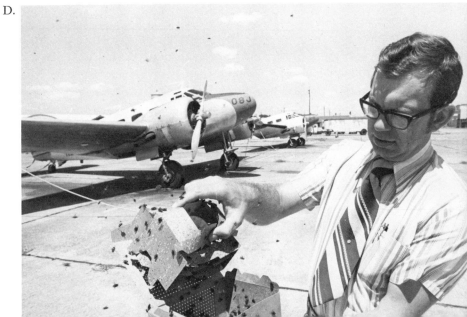

waters to a reasonable ecological state. For example, concerted action over the last decade has greatly reduced pollution in San Diego Bay and in Seattle's Lake Washington.

PESTS

Most pesticides are *broad-spectrum* poisons; that is, they harm many organisms in addition to their intended targets. Most are also long-lasting. Attempts are being made to develop new and improved pesticides which will affect only their target species and which will break down into harmless substances soon after application.

BETTER LIVING THROUGH LESS TECHNOLOGY:

3. PEST CONTROL

Some biologists feel we have placed too much emphasis on fighting pests, that an ecologically sounder approach would be to reduce controls and let our crops come into balance with their pests. The resulting crop losses could be offset by increasing the number of acres planted. One estimate is that a 70 to 80 per cent reduction in insecticides could be offset by a 12 per cent increase in crop land.

There is some support for the idea that we have overreacted to certain pests. The fire ant, for example, has been the subject of a large-scale eradication program that may turn out to be largely a waste of time. The fire ant was carried into this country from South America around fifty years ago and is now well established in the Southeast. Fire ants build rather large mounds in open fields, and as their name implies, they have a somewhat nasty sting. Numerous reports and articles describe the fire ant as a major pest. As one such article said, "A formidable army of South American fire ants has invaded the United States. . . . Already the destructive insects have captured much of the South's best farmland and are eating their way northward and westward. Their onslaught, if unchecked, may not stop short of California and Canada." [19] The fire ant is cited as killing newborn farm animals, causing widespread damage to crops, attacking man without provocation, and causing damage to harvesting machinery because of its mounds. As a result, extensive control measures have been initiated, particularly by the United States Department of Agriculture. The

Although synthetic pesticides probably will remain the major weapon against pests, another approach is to try to make living things do the job. The most successful example of this is the work of Edward Knipling, now director of entomology research in the Agricultural Research Service of the United States Department of Agriculture. For many years, the screw worm fly was a dangerous pest of American cattle and swine. The adult fly lays its eggs in the open sores or wounds which domestic animals sometimes have, and the hatching larvae then burrow into the animal's flesh. About twenty-five years ago, Knipling theorized that the screw worm fly might be controlled if large numbers of male flies were sterilized and then released. These

insecticide of choice since 1962 has been Mirex, a chlorinated hydrocarbon.

Actually, it seems that the fire ant is overrated as a pest. Various laboratory and field studies suggest that it does not commonly attack animals and crops, and, at least in its natural habitat, the fire ant is beneficial as a controller of other insects. Furthermore, the sting of the fire ant is really no more of a problem than a wasp or bee sting. On the other hand, Mirex acts as do DDT and other chlorinated hydrocarbons. There is evidence that it accumulates in food chains, becoming concentrated in such valuable resources as the oysters and shellfish of the Gulf Coast. In short, it may be that the cure is worse than the pest—especially since Mirex so far has failed to halt the fire ant's spread.

Fire ant mounds in Louisiana. (USDA photo.)

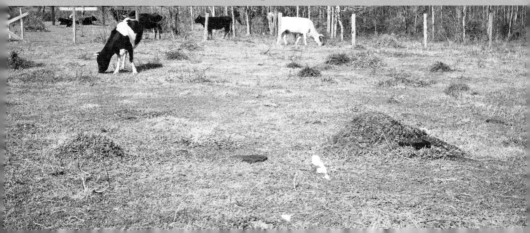

males would mate with females and the females would then produce unfertile eggs. Since a female fly mates only once, the effect would be to drastically reduce the size of the next generation. In the early 1950's Knipling finally was able to test his idea. Thousands of flies were exposed to X-rays. The rays broke chromosomes in the flies' gonads, so that the flies produced sterile sperm. These sterile flies then were released on Sanibel Island off the coast of Florida, an area of heavy screw worm infestation. The local population of flies decreased, but new flies promptly migrated from the mainland.

One day, Knipling received a letter from a veterinarian on the Caribbean island of Curaçao, asking for ideas about controlling the screw worm fly. Knipling's response was to shift his whole operation there, for Curaçao is small and isolated, and so provided an ideal spot to test his scheme. With the cooperation of the local government, 150,000 sterile flies were released each week in the summer of 1954. After three months, the local screw worm fly population was eradicated.

Knipling then set up a massive operation in Florida. In eighteen months, over 2½ billion sterile males were released from airplanes. By 1958, the screw worm fly was eliminated from Florida. Texas was next, and with the success of the program there, the pest was effectively eliminated from the United States. Our government now maintains a control zone along the Mexican border, and plans call for an expansion of the program into that country.

Knipling's program has two great ecological advantages over the use of pesticides. First, it is hard to think of any mutation which would make the screw worm resistant to the program, and second, other organisms are not harmed. Knipling's technique is being tried with certain other pests whose behavior patterns make them subject to this kind of biological control.

Another method of biological control is to import foreign insects or other organisms, which then act as parasites or predators of some domestic pest. This can be a bit tricky, for the introduced species will sometimes change their ways and become pests themselves. For example, Glover Allen tells what happened when the mongoose was introduced into Jamaica to control rats. "In 1872, W. Bancroft Espeut imported four pairs of mongoose from Calcutta to Jamaica, for the purpose of destroying the rats that caused so great a destruction of sugar cane. These four pairs increased so rapidly, and attacked the rats with such ardor, that ten years later it was estimated that they effected an annual saving to the colony of 100,000 pounds sterling.

Shortly after, however, they had so reduced the rats that they fell upon the native ground animals and nearly annihilated certain toads, lizards, birds, and mammals." [20]

Some more exotic means of pest control are available or are being developed. Many insects go through a complex series of molts, which are controlled by growth hormones. These hormones can be synthesized and used as insecticides, for they will cause an insect to molt at abnormal times or in abnormal ways and so fail to reproduce. Some insects produce chemicals which act as sex attractants, and these can be used to lure the unsuspecting pest to his death.

Our technology has developed or proposed many solutions for our ecological crisis. However, if these are to work at all, we must first make some decisions about Western technology itself. Since our technology created the ecological crisis, is it realistic to assume that more of the same technology can solve it? If we decide in the affirmative, will we find ourselves eventually living in a sterile technological environment in which all human values have been lost?

Before attacking these questions, we will first consider what Western technology has done to the health of man.

13 MAN'S HEALTH: PROGRESS

THE CONQUEST OF INFECTIOUS DISEASE

Cholera is a terrifying disease. It begins with a feeling of vague fullness of the abdomen and a loss of appetite. This is followed by dizziness, clammy extremities, repeated vomiting, and abdominal cramps painful enough to double the victim up in agony. The most characteristic symptom is the appearance of so-called rice-water diarrhea, a copious, watery fluid containing portions of the victim's intestinal wall. Cholera victims lose up to a liter of liquid per hour in diarrhea. Over many hours as much as a fourth of one's body weight is lost. After days of misery the cholera victim will slowly recover or more commonly will die. The incidence of death in untreated cases runs between 50 and 70 per cent.

Cholera has been an endemic disease in Asia, particularly in India, for thousands of years. For little-understood reasons it occasionally breaks out and sweeps across new territory as a global epidemic or pandemic. Asiatic cholera first reached the United States in pandemic form in 1832. Its arrival was not unexpected, for its progress across Europe had been watched with increasing anxiety by Americans. Leaving India in 1816, it was in Moscow by 1830 and in western Europe by 1831. In 1832 it appeared in the New World, first in Quebec, then in New York and Philadelphia, and finally in the Midwest.

161

What could American medicine of the 1830's do to manage this dread disease? Some doctors thought the disease was caused by tiny insects or *animalculae* in the air, but no such contagious agent could be identified. Most thought a variety of factors probably caused the disease. A lack of personal cleanliness, bad diet, excessive exercise, sitting in the sun or in an air current, miasmas or unhealthy mists, and even a high ground-water level were all cited as contributing agents. Ideas about prevention were as varied as supposed causes. Dr. Daniel Drake of Cincinnati, probably the best-known doctor in the Midwest, advised his patients to maintain a calm mind and wear thin flannels. Treatments included a variety of medications. Opium and calomel (which contains mercury and in any volume is poisonous) were prescribed. One widely used medication was concocted of West Indian rum, molasses, and certain herbs, such as lobelia and pepper. Patients sometimes were bled.

Cholera remained a dread disease, resisting all attempts at treatment, until the full power of science coupled with technology could be brought to bear on it. A major breakthrough in the understanding of cholera took place in the 1850's. During the English cholera epidemic of 1854, John Snow, a London doctor, noticed that in one part of the city a suspicious number of cholera cases cropped up among people who had at least one habit in common—they all shared a neighborhood water pump (Figure 13-1). Guessing that something in the water supply caused cholera, Snow had the pump overseers remove the handle so that the pump could not be used, and neighborhood cases of cholera promptly decreased.

Snow's hypothesis that cholera was caused by some water-borne agent was confirmed by Robert Koch in the 1880's. Both Koch and Louis Pasteur, the great French microbiologist, had been successfully identifying disease organisms for a decade and both were certain a cholera microbe could be found. As bitter rivals, each tried to scoop the other and find the hypothesized agent first. Both were frustrated by the lack of cholera patients in Europe at the time. Koch, however, went to India and found the cholera microbe, identifying its presence in victims who had died of cholera, in their soiled linen, and even in the water tanks of Indian villages. Although a causative agent for cholera had now been found, there were still some skeptics. Max Pettenkofer, the scientist who had thought high water levels caused cholera, asked Koch to send him some of his so-called cholera germs. Koch did, and Pettenkofer swallowed enough to infect an army—without any ill effects!

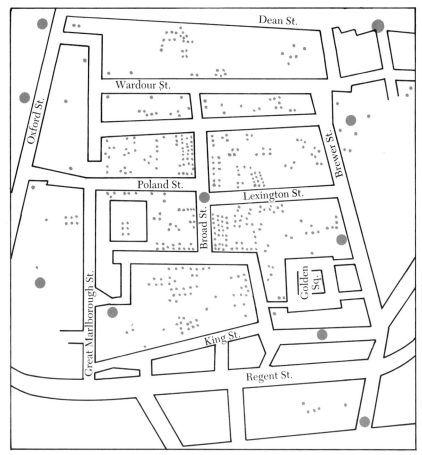

Figure 13-1. Map of the Soho district of London. Large dots mark drinking-water pumps. Small dots mark houses where cholera occurred in epidemic of 1854. When Broad Street pump was put out of use, cholera dropped sharply in the district.

Continued research on the causes for cholera uncovered the fact that it could be spread by routes other than water. Some people were found to be *carriers*. Although cured of the disease and free of any symptoms, they continued to harbor the microbe, shedding it into food or other materials with which they came into contact.

During the nineteenth century, a whole series of other infectious diseases came under scientific investigation. In addition to cholera, these included typhus, malaria, typhoid fever, smallpox, and tuberculosis. Armed with the understanding provided by science, doctors slowly began to develop effective treatments against infectious disease.

The most significant gains against infectious disease, however, did not come from medical science, but were associated with a slowly rising standard of living in the Western world. Many of these advances began to appear well before the nature of infectious disease was understood. Sanitary water supply systems were developed. Cess pits and open drains were replaced with sewage systems. Housing legislation removed the worst offenses in urban slum areas. Other legislation led to control over the processing of food. Mass production, for example, led to disposable paper cups, a much more effective barrier to waterborne disease than the old-fashioned drinking cup. Packaging techniques allowed food to escape handling or contamination by pests. Mechanized agricultural technology drained swamplands which formerly housed mosquitoes, the carriers of malaria and yellow fever. House screens furthered this protection, as did insecticides. The very construction materials increasingly used in Western technology—

THE COUNTRY DOCTOR (Circa 1830)

The equipment of a typical country doctor was simple. Often he made his rounds on horseback, carrying his instruments in saddlebags. Much of his diagnosis depended on long experience—he relied more on a feel for sickness, how a patient looked and acted, the color of his skin, his temperature, or the appearance of his tongue than he did on any instruments. His instruments might include a stethoscope, forceps to extract teeth, obstetrical devices, and a diagnostic instrument called a pulsometer. This was hourglass shaped and contained a colored liquid. The patient held one end and could see bubbles rise in the other. Pulsometers told nothing about the patient's condition, but they were impressive and helped convince the sick person that his doctor was doing something about his illness. Almost all doctors carried some kind of lancet, which was used to treat fevers by drawing blood. Some varieties resembled a pocket knife; others had a kind of spring attachment, so the blade would penetrate to a set depth. Patients were often bled until they were faint, after which they might be given an emetic or perhaps an opium compound. Other rough treatments included immersion in hot or cold water for the ague, as the ever-present malaria was called. Still other treatments used a moxa or a seton. A moxa was a

metals, glass, and plastics—proved easier to keep sanitized. Railroad and household refrigeration protected food from decay and contamination.

Along with his increasing affluence, Western man developed an aversion to dirt. Daily bathing and the washing of hands before meals slowly became the rule. Table etiquette itself changed drastically. We no longer accepted the medieval practice of using hands instead of forks at table or of dipping our fingers into a common pot, licking them clean, and returning for more. The presence of rats, lice, and fleas became thought of as repulsive rather than as a part of living. Widespread and efficient communication systems alerted communities to potential epidemics so they could prepare defenses. Better nutritional practices resulted in an increased ability to fight off potential infections. All of these things were at once part of and a consequence of a new technology which could produce a higher standard of living.

coil of cotton, treated so that it would burn slowly when placed on the skin, and thus raise a blister. A seton was a thread placed in a cut or wound to inflame or "create an issue."

However bizarre these treatments might appear, they were nevertheless derived from a rational theory of the cause of disease. This was the theory that sickness results from an upset of harmony or balance in body fluids. The concept itself went back to the Aristotelian view of nature as composed of four elements: earth, air, fire, and water. To many Greek thinkers our body contained four comparable elements or *humors*: blood, yellow bile, black bile, and phlegm. An upset in the balance of these humors was thought to cause disease. We have not quite abandoned this idea, for we still talk about being phlegmatic, bilious, or in a bad humor. While the country doctor did not think of his treatments as Aristotelian, they were an outgrowth of this view. Thus he drew blood to reduce an excess of humor or blistered with a moxa to stir up the body and restore deficiency of some humor. Oddly enough, in what we hope is a more sophisticated way, in modern environmental medicine we tend to revive the idea that health is harmony or balance and disease, a loss of these qualities.

Coupled with the advances of medical science, this new pattern of living has effectively banished most of the great infectious diseases from the Western nations.

THE RISE OF MODERN SURGERY

Evidence from skeletons suggests that hunting-gathering man did on occasion resort to surgery to combat real or imagined sickness. Attempts were probably made to reduce fractures. Trephination, an operation in which the skull was opened, seems to have been practiced by many peoples. It may have been in response either to concussion or to brain damage, but it may also have been carried out in connection with religious rites. At any rate, even if narcotics were available it must have been an exceedingly dangerous and painful experience.

Before the advent of modern medical science and technology, Western surgery was not much different. It also was a hazardous, unpleasant experience and a last-resort treatment. Anesthetics, for

Figure 13-2. Unlike hunting-gathering man, urban man cannot easily escape his disease-producing refuse. Varick Street, New York, late in the 19th century. (Photograph by Jacob A. Riis. Courtesy of the Jacob A. Riis Collection, Museum of the City of New York.)

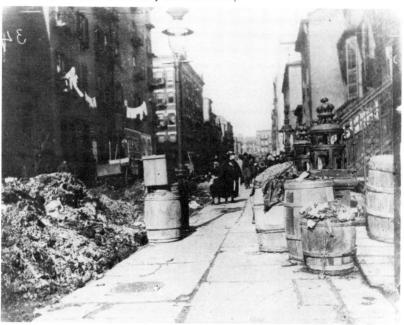

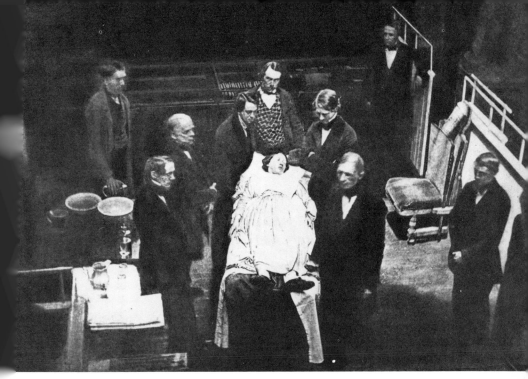

Figure 13-3. An operation at Massachusetts General Hospital in 1847. The surgeon is using ether, which had been introduced the year before. Note street dress of attending physicians. (Courtesy of the National Library of Medicine.)

Figure 13-4. Illustration from text of 1882, showing use of Lister's carbolic acid spray. (Courtesy of the National Library of Medicine.)

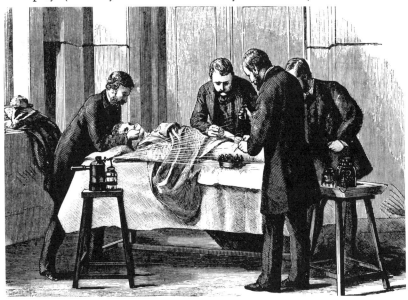

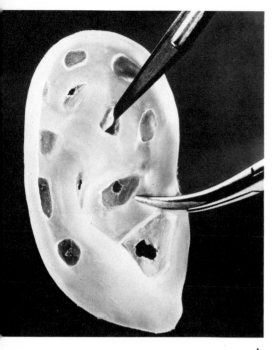

A.

Figure 13-5. Surgical implants made of silicone. A. An ear implant. B, C. Before and after photographs of a recipient. D. A finger joint designed by Dr. A. B. Swanson of Grand Rapids, Michigan. E, F. Before and after surgery. (Photographs courtesy of Dow Corning Corporation, Midland, Michigan.)

D.

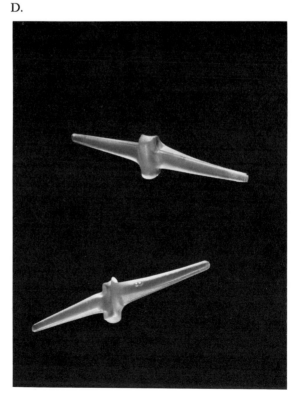

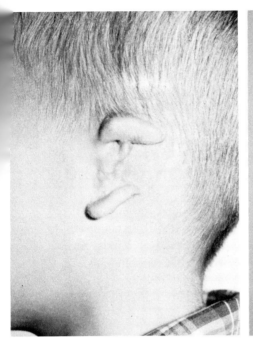

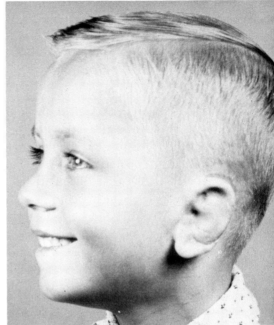

B.

C.

E.

F.

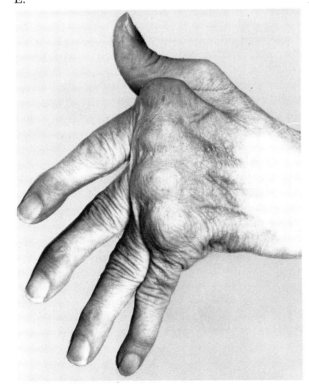

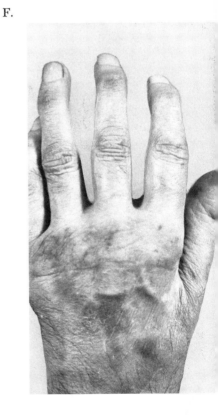

example, did not come into general use until after the 1840's. Before then, a patient for surgery might get himself drunk or otherwise prepare himself for the ordeal. Some doctors had tried hypnotizing their patients, but generally surgery was an agonizing ordeal. As a result, speed was of the utmost importance. Some of the most skilled surgeons of the time could take off a leg in less than a minute. Unfortunately, since nothing was known about the nature of infection, no attempt was made to sterilize the surgeon, his operating instruments, or the patient. The surgeon would often work in an old blood-encrusted overcoat or operating grown. Ligatures to suture the wound would be pinned to the coat. Blood would be wiped from the wound with a damp sponge which would be rinsed in water and reused until it fell apart. Medical students sometimes went directly from autopsies to assist in an operation, never bothering to wash their hands. As one surgeon of the time put it, "no one dreamed of washing his hands before an operation; one washed them afterwards." [21]

Under these conditions, post-operative mortality was extremely high, particularly when need arose to enter the abdomen or thoracic cavity. All this changed rapidly with the advent of the germ theory of disease. Although others—particularly the American Oliver Wendell Holmes and the Viennese obstetrician Ignaz Semmelweiss—had pointed the way, Joseph Lister, a London surgeon, usually is credited with showing conclusively that the germs in the dirt surrounding an operation were the cause of infection. When Lister read of Pasteur's work with microbes, he immediately associated them with surgical infections and developed a technique of spraying the operating room, patient, surgeons, and surgical instruments with carbolic acid, an antiseptic (Figure 13-4). Many doctors ridiculed Lister. Even in the 1870's it was still a common joke between English surgeons to shout at anyone who appeared in the doorway of the operating theatre, "Shut that door quickly, otherwise you'll let Lister's microbes in!" [22] In spite of ridicule, the system worked, and with the Lister technique, mortality rates after surgery dropped dramatically.

After Lister, many surgeons rejected his *antisepsis* technique in favor of *asepsis*. Instead of trying to massacre all the germs in the vicinity, the doctors eliminated them through a strict regimen of asepsis, prior removal by washing and sterilizing. Asepsis is still a basic part of operative technique. Anesthetics, antiseptics, and asepsis produced a revolution in surgery, for the way was now open to develop a variety of new operative techniques.

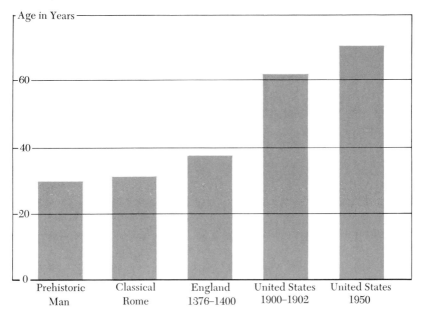

Figure 13-6. Longevity in ancient and modern times. (After Deevey, E. S., Jr., "The Human Population," *Scientific American*, 203, September 1960, pp. 194–204.)

All sorts of sophisticated procedures have now become routine. One of the most striking accomplishments of modern surgery is its ability to use artificial materials as replacement parts for damaged or diseased organs. Figure 13-5 indicates one common surgical technique —the replacement of faulty parts with silicone implants.

With his relatively weak technology, hunting-gathering man could do little to protect himself from the effects of disease. As a result, he rarely lived a long life. Western medical technology finally has broken the hold of disease, and as a result Western man enjoys an average life expectancy far above that of his ancestors (Figure 13-6).

14 HEALTH PROBLEMS CREATED BY WESTERN TECHNOLOGY

In spite of his technology and its great power, complete health still eludes Western man. Surprisingly enough, some would argue that technology has not increased our state of health at all, but actually lowered it. Organic diseases, for example, particularly cancer and the cardiovascular diseases, have risen from a relatively minor position on the disease list and are now our major health concerns.

Automobile accidents are also now one of our major health problems. Over one and a half million people have died since this particular kind of epidemic began in 1899, when a Mr. Bliss stepped off a trolley car in New York City and was hit by one of the new "horseless carriages." Other accidents, both at work and in the home, are also a major health problem.

A whole spectrum of genetic diseases such as cystic fibrosis and sickle cell anemia, which no one had even heard of a hundred years ago, now are recognized as major health concerns. Finally, while most infectious diseases are coming under the control of modern medical technology, none has been eradicated and some, such as salmonellosis and serum hepatitis, actually have increased in frequency. Why is it that we seem to be treading water or even losing ground as far as our health is concerned?

It has been a repeated theme of this book that in the Western world cultural evolution has created a new kind of environment, different

Death Rate per
100,000 of Population

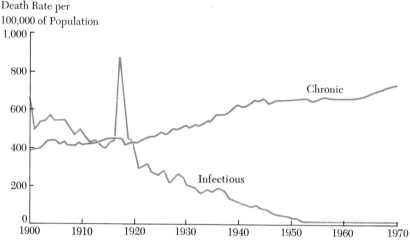

Figure 14-1. The shift in America from infectious to chronic organic diseases, especially the cardiovascular diseases and cancer. (After Glazier, W. H., "The Task of Medicine," *Scientific American*, 228, April 1973, pp. 13–17.

from that in which all life, including man, evolved. Six key characteristics of this new environment can be directly implicated as causes of Western man's health problems. These are a new kind of stress, the mechanization of our environment, toxic materials, overnutrition, the human monoculture, and the technological shield.

A NEW KIND OF STRESS

As was suggested in Chapter 1, all living things, including man, are designed to exist in a homeostatic or steady state. The term *stress* can be defined as any environmental stimulus which acts to upset this state of equilibrium. Since man lives in a continually changing environment and routinely encounters new and unanticipated situations, he is under a continuous state of stress. Some situations, as when we are caught in a sudden downpour, trip over a rock, run for a bus, or receive a mediocre grade on a test, produce a relatively mild state of stress. Others, perhaps an encounter with a psychopathic killer or becoming ill with cholera, produce much greater stress.

Over millions of years, our bodies have evolved a complex stress system which responds to all stressful stimuli, whether large or small. The *hypothalamus*, which lies at the base of the brain, forms the heart of this system. It receives incoming stressful stimuli, coordinates these, and then sends messages to various organ systems, instructing them to carry out an appropriate response to the stress. Some of these messages go via our nervous system, others by way of hormones in the blood-stream.

A stressful situation can trigger a wide range of bodily responses. Your heart may pound, your stomach churn, and your pupils dilate. Many of the body's responses to stress are not obvious. The blood vessels in your muscles may dilate and the glucose level in your blood may rise. Studies have even shown that the chemistry of your urine will change. All of these bodily changes act to prepare you to cope with the stress situation you face. Over most of man's evolutionary history, almost all stress situations have involved some physical threat. For this reason, your body responds to stress by alerting you and preparing you for physical action. Thus, the stress response is sometimes called the *fight or flight syndrome.*

If these reactions were to continue for too long a period or become too widespread, the body's tissues would be severely damaged, and death would result. Therefore, a very important segment of the stress system acts as a moderator, dampening down, localizing, and generally helping to cushion the primary stress response. This is done through the action of the *cortisols,* hormones produced by the adrenal glands.

Environmental stimuli, and the inevitable stresses which accompany them, are a basic part of life, and without them we would not be human. As one author has put it:

> Whether we think we like it or not, it is quite probable that the healthy human psyche requires a proportion of roughage in its figurative diet. We are the heirs of a million years of a generally victorious struggle against cold, hunger, difficult terrain, carnivorous cunning; our nervous and glandular balance has evolved under the stress of exertion, effort, endurance. Individuals reared in the complete absence of such stimuli are not apt to be healthy or sane.[23]

This point is borne out by experiments in which college students were placed in lukewarm water, given darkened goggles to wear, and kept in a room in which the only noise they heard was a steady hum. Although the students thought that their stay might provide them with a chance to relax and catch up on their thinking, they ended up having hallucinations and other abnormal perceptive reactions.

If stress is a normal and even desirable component of life, why is it a problem in our technological environment? To answer this, it is necessary to look at the nature of stress under Western technology. Our type of stress differs from that which hunting-gathering man encountered in three fundamental ways.

Anticipatory Stress—The Price of a Future-Oriented Society

Almost certainly, hunting-gathering men worried. Yet, as we noted in Chapter 6, hunting-gathering peoples tend to take life on a day-to-day basis and to Western man appear almost apathetic. In contrast, we live in a future-oriented culture. As a result, we are immersed constantly in a flood of anticipatory worries. What will we do on the next test? What will the job be like? What does the future hold for us?

Of course, these stresses are all imagined. Yet, the body's stress system reacts to them in exactly the same way as it does to immediate physical stress. This is so because over its long evolution, the body has been programmed for stresses that were overwhelmingly physical in nature and it knows of no other way to respond.

Concern over a wide variety of coming events will produce a stress reaction in the body. Worrying about a coming speech, acting as coxswain of a racing shell, trying to meet a term paper deadline, or even waiting for the next scene in a violent movie will do this. There is no adaptive value in preparing the body for fight or flight in situations of this sort, but the stress system is automatic and we have no way of turning it off. In effect, then, our anxiety-ridden, future-oriented society has produced an entirely new set of stressful events with which our bodies must cope.

New Kinds of Physical Stress

Modern man makes his way through a maze of neon lights, listens to loud rock music, becomes disoriented from the time change of a long flight, sits cramped at a desk all day long, and drives at seventy miles an hour on a crowded expressway. He sees these stressful situations as a normal part of his life style. To his body, however, they are novel challenges, for which it was not evolved. After all, we are designed to travel around three miles per hour and certainly not to move across time zones. Nor were our senses designed to process the kaleidoscopic variety of our urban scene, or the decibel level of rock music. Thus, modern man is subject not only to the anticipatory stress of a future-oriented society, but also to a variety of new physical stresses unknown to his ancestors.

The Variety of Stress in a Changing Society

As Toffler has documented so well in his book *Future Shock*, we live in a throw-away society in which everything we do or use or even believe is geared to change. Somewhere around forty million Americans will move this year, a far higher percentage than in any other country except perhaps Canada. The average American moves fourteen times in his lifetime. As Vance Packard says in the title of his book, we are a *Nation of Strangers*, rootless and without a sense of place. As twentieth-century nomads, we are continually subject to new and changing environments and thus to new and changing stresses.

Stress and Disease

What happens when a stress system which was evolved to cope with the relatively benign environment of a hunting-gathering world is placed within our more complex technological world, with its new levels of stress? Many scientists think that this can easily create an overload of the stress system. Although the exact mechanisms are not understood, overloading the stress system seems to throw it out of balance. This in turn disrupts its target organs, leading to organic disease. Is there any evidence to link a particularly stressful life style with organic disease? A number of studies have suggested such a link. Here are four examples:

1. *The heart-attack type.* Dr. Meyer Friedman of San Francisco has spent fifteen years studying the medical histories of three thousand San Francisco men in an attempt to see if there is any such thing as a heart-attack-prone personality. He has found that people who are excessively ambitious, aggressive, impatient, and slaves to the clock have two and a half times as many heart attacks as do quieter, more relaxed people. His heart attack personality profile is also a classic profile of someone who is excessively subject to stress.

2. *Black hypertension.* High blood pressure or hypertension is more than twice as common among blacks in this country as among whites. Present estimates are that one of every seven blacks has high blood pressure, and some researchers think the figure is actually closer to one in four. Furthermore, blacks begin to show high blood pressure earlier than whites and it is often more severe. This difference is largely found among poorer ghetto people rather than among middle-class blacks.

Psychologists have theorized that when anger or frustration has no outlet, it will become internalized and lead to high levels of mental

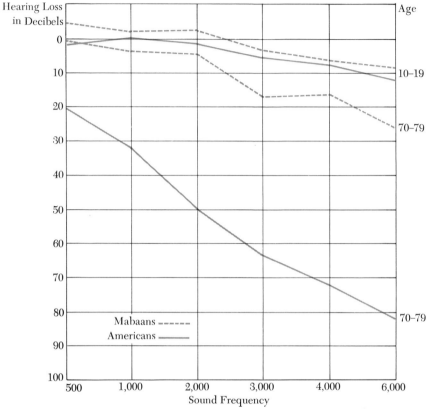

Figure 14-2. Hearing loss in Mabaans and Americans. By the time they reach old age, Americans differ significantly from the Mabaans in their ability to hear higher frequency sounds. (Data from Rosen, S., and P. Olin, "Hearing Loss and Coronary Heart Disease," *Archives of Otolaryngology,* 82: 236, 1965, as given in Benarde, Melvin A., *Our Precarious Habitat,* New York: W.W. Norton & Company, Inc., 1970.)

stress. The inability of poorer blacks to get ahead in a white society may lead to just this sort of frustration, producing excessive stress, which in turn causes hypertension.

3. *The hearing ability of Maabans and Americans.* The Maabans are primitive villagers who live in the Egyptian Sudan. Compared to Americans, older Maabans show very little hearing loss (Figure 14-2). On first examination, this difference would seem a direct result of the auditory pounding our ears take. Actually, the cause-effect pathway may be somewhat more involved. Unlike the Maabans, Americans live in a stress-ridden society. This contributes to our high incidence of

hypertension, which is a rare disease among the Maabans. Hypertension, in turn, damages our inner ear, thus leading to hearing loss among older Americans.

4. *Life-change units.* Perhaps the most interesting work associating disease with excessive stress is that which has utilized a research tool called the *Life-Change Units Scale.* The researchers involved in this study began with a list of various stressful situations such as divorce, death of spouse, moving, losing a job, and preparing for a vacation. Thousands of informants were asked to rank these stressful situations according to their relative severity. By averaging the responses, each situation was given a relative weight and a Life-Change Units Scale was compiled. Death of one's spouse, for example, received a hundred points; moving to a new home received twenty. The researchers then went to a second group of subjects and compiled their life-change scores over a set period of time. Finally, they checked the health of these subjects during the same period. Their findings showed a strong positive correlation: The greater the life change score, the greater the amount of sickness. The diseases recorded were of a wide variety. Their conclusion: When the stress associated with our culture's high rate of variation and change becomes too great, our stress mechanism somehow malfunctions, and the result is disease.

THE MECHANIZATION OF OUR ENVIRONMENT

Mechanization Takes Command

In an earlier chapter we characterized hunting-gathering cultures as hand-powered. With his hand-powered tools, primitive man lacked the capacity to transform the environment radically. In contrast, our machine-powered culture has been able to create an artificial, mechanized environment. Stop a moment and look at the objects which surround you. Most likely, they have one or more of the following characteristics.

1. They are hard, smooth, angular. Many natural objects also have these qualities, but they are much more pronounced in our machine environment. After all, steel beams, waxed floors, and razor blades are rare in nature.

2. Many of the objects surrounding us are self-powered. Washing machines, foundry presses, and household fans move in the absence of any human hand to direct them. Even when a human is present, as in the case of cars or airplanes, our powered objects have a surprising

degree of independence and can easily get away from their human masters. We have come to be more or less used to our menagerie of independent or semi-independent machines and forget that nothing comparable exists in nature.

3. Many objects in our environment are loaded with latent power. High-tension wires or a stick of dynamite are examples.

Mechanization and Disease

Many of our accidents are of course similar to those which befell hunting-gathering man. However, an increasing percentage of our mishaps are of a new kind. These are the accidents which are a consequence of the three characteristics of a mechanized environment which we have just listed, characteristics with which our bodies were never evolved to cope.

If we were to choose the typical accident of modern man, it would be the automobile accident. If rates continue as in the present, every other American will either be killed or injured in an auto accident at some time during his life. Although a vast literature exists on the causes of automobile accidents and huge amounts of money are expended on driver-education programs, there is no way that we can be taught to surmount the fundamental problem involved. The human body was simply not designed to cope with a semi-autonomous machine which is built of hard, angular metal and moves at rates of thirty to seventy miles per hour.

Household accidents also reflect the body's lack of adaptation to a mechanized environment. Every year home accidents injure twenty million and kill thirty thousand. Some of the greatest hazards are glass windows, walls, and doors; kitchen equipment; and bathrooms; particularly slippery tub floors. As our home technologies change, new hazards arise. Power-mower accidents, almost unknown twenty years ago, are a good example of this.

TOXIC MATERIALS

Toxic Materials In Our Environment

Man has always encountered toxic materials in his environment. Poisonous plants and animals, bad water, and other similar hazards must have taken their toll among hunting-gathering peoples.

Our Western technological environment, however, differs from all previous environments in the number and magnitude of toxic substances it contains. As a result of our power to manipulate nature, we busily produce thousands of new and potentially toxic compounds or concentrate others which once were dispersed or rare in nature.

A rather large body of evidence exists which suggests that these substances which man's body never was adapted to deal with may have much to do with the rise of organic disease in the Western world today.

Toxic Materials and Cancer

A vast literature has accumulated dealing with the possibility that many substances produced by Western technology are *carcinogenic*, that is, cancer-inducing. Weed and insect killers, food preservatives and other food additives, cigarette smoke and other air pollutants, plastics which give off fumes, industrial chemicals, and various kinds of radiation have all been implicated. It is generally agreed that in the aggregate, our technological environment has more carcinogenic substances than did earlier ones and that this fact certainly accounts, in part at least, for the prevalence of cancer today.

Here are a few examples of substances which have either been shown to have or are suspected to have carcinogenic activity. Many additional ones could be cited.

1. *M.G.A.* Our food contains a huge number of synthetic materials. Some, such as the cyclamates, which until recently were used as artificial sweeteners, have been implicated as potential carcinogens and banned from use. Others are only suspect. One of these is M.G.A., a rather interesting material because of the way it becomes incorporated into our food.

M.G.A., or melengestrol acetate, is a synthetic hormone used by operators of cattle feed lots. Mixed into the food of female beef cattle, M.G.A. supresses their reproductive cycle, which relaxes them and quickens their weight gain. M.G.A. concentrates in the tissues of cattle and so passes on to our tables. The Food and Drug Administration considers M.G.A. a suspected carcinogen, but has not as yet banned its use.

2. *Asbestos.* Manville, New Jersey, is a town of fifteen thousand. Its largest source of income is the Johns-Manville Company, where two thousand of the townspeople work. Johns-Manville is the largest manufacturer of asbestos products in this country. Asbestos is used in at least three thousand products, including theatre curtains, drapes, potholders, ironing boards, floor tiling, wallboard, brake linings, and mufflers. If the reader has ever worked with asbestos, he will know

how it has a way of getting into or onto everything, particularly those places where it is not wanted. Needless to say, the residents of Manville, particularly the plant workers, are exposed to large amounts of asbestos. In Manville lung cancer is four times as common as in the nation at large. In the last eight years, fifty-eight people in Manville have contracted mesothelioma, a rather rare type of chest or abdominal cancer. The conclusion is inescapable—asbestos acts as a carcinogen. This is a particularly difficult realization for Manville residents to face. Cancers often have a long latent period. That of mesothelioma, for example, is probably twenty to forty years. As a result, even though strong steps will now be taken, many Manville residents already must be on their way to developing cancer.

3. *Air pollution.* The epidemiology of cancer is a very complex subject, particularly since so many agents have been suspected as carcinogens. One special type of air pollutant, cigarette smoke, has been established thoroughly as a prime cause of lung cancer, and other air pollutants are also under suspicion. This suspicion is based on the finding that urban living seems to predispose a person to lung cancer, and the longer one lives in the city, the greater are his chances of getting the disease. In one study of 2,191 lung cancer deaths among males, the urban death rate was almost one and a half times that of rural areas. Among those who had lived in the city all their lives, the incidence was twice as great. Almost all of those who are involved in the epidemiology of cancer think the key carcinogenic factor in urban areas is air pollution.

4. *Radiation.* It is a well-known fact that radiation can cause cancer, particularly those cancers collectively called the leukemias. There is some evidence that radiation also causes thyroid, lung, and breast cancer. Although we sometimes act as if it were a new phenomenon, man has always been subjected to radiation. Some of this natural radiation comes from cosmic sources, some from minerals within the earth. While radiation is not new to man, modern industrial and medical technology is rapidly creating new sources of radiation. This raises a key question. At what point are the benefits derived from the activities associated with this new radiation outweighed by its hazard to our lives? In this country the Federal Radiation Council (since absorbed into the Environmental Protection Agency) has established a permissible level of 170 millirems ° of industrial radiation a year. This

° A rem is defined as the deposition in tissue of one hundred ergs of energy. A millirem is one-thousandth of a rem.

Table 14-1. *Radiation Received Annually by Typical American*

Source of radiation	Dose in millirems per year
Environmental	
Natural sources	102
Global fallout	4
Nuclear power	0.003
Subtotal	106
Medical	
Diagnostic	72
Drugs	1
Subtotal	73
Other	3
Total	182

From Robert Gillette, "Radiation Standards: The Last Word or at Least a Definitive One," *Science*, **178**, December 1, 1972, p. 966 ff.

would be in addition to the roughly 180 millirems we now receive each year from medical and natural sources. The 170 figure essentially sanctioned a continuing expansion of industrial radiation, which is now at a negligible level (Table 14-1). What would happen if overall radiation should increase by 170 millirems or more? Opinions vary. A National Academy of Science committee has estimated that it would ultimately create 6,000 additional cancer deaths per year. Other estimates range upward to 32,000 deaths a year. In the meantime, radiation levels produced by medical and industrial technology are rising, year by year.

Toxic Materials and Cardiovascular Disease

Just as with cancer, a variety of toxic materials seem to contribute to cardiovascular disease. Air pollution has at least an indirect effect, since anything that puts a strain on the lungs will do the same for the heart. Strong links have been established between smoking and heart disease. Interestingly enough, women are catching up with men in coronary disease, which may be a reflection of the rise in women smokers over the last two decades. Industrial chemicals also have been implicated. A survey of twenty-eight cities in the United States showed a good correlation between cadmium in the environment and deaths from high blood pressure and heart disease.

Most interest, however, focuses on the role of diet in causing cardiovascular disease. We don't think of it in that way, but when viewed in evolutionary terms, Western man's diet is unnatural and thus potentially toxic. Americans eat much more fat than primitive man ever did (the Eskimo and Masai are exceptions to this), and we also eat more sugar than did primitives. Our diet is particularly rich in items such as fat-marbled steaks, ice cream, cheese, chocolate bars, and butter. All of these contain cholesterol, a colorless, odorless material. Animal fats, particularly saturated ones composed of long chain molecules, and cholesterol have come to be regarded as prime culprits in the rise of cardiovascular disease among modern Western man. Evidence for this has been accumulating steadily from studies made over the last twenty years.

Some of these studies have compared the incidence of heart disease in different cultures. The South African Bantu, for example, receive only 17 per cent of their caloric intake from fats as compared to our 40 to 50 per cent, and their coronary rate is far below ours. Over the last twenty years the Japanese diet has shifted steadily from rice, fish, and vegetables toward a Western one heavy in fat. During this period their death rate from strokes, coronaries, and other arterial failures has doubled.

Other studies have compared different groups of Americans. One of the best designed of these was carried out on 850 elderly men at a Veterans Hospital in Los Angeles. The men were divided randomly into two groups. One group ate the hospital's usual food, which contained appreciable amounts of saturated fats. The other group ate food cooked with a minimum of fat, which, when used, was unsaturated. The subjects did not know which kind of food they were eating. During the study, thirteen of those on a low-fat diet died of heart disease, while thirty-one in the other group died. Other, larger studies have shown approximately the same results. One imaginative study has compared heart attack rates in different Catholic orders. Trappist monks, who exist on a Spartan diet, have ninety heart attacks per 100,000 man years, a very low figure. Trappist fathers, who enjoy a richer diet, have 290. Benedictine monks, members of a more permissive order, also have a rate of 290. Benedictine fathers, who enjoy a very rich diet, have 920 attacks per 100,000 man years.

Somehow, a high-fat diet seems to be associated with the deposit on artery walls of lipoprotein *plaques*, which contain cholesterol and other fatty materials. Through a process not completely understood, these deposits gradually thicken on the arterial walls until circulation

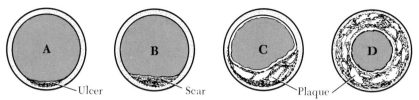

Figure 14-3. Plaque deposits in arteries. A. Ulcer develops on inner surface of artery. B. Scar tissue forms over ulcer. C. Plaques composed of cholesterol, lipoprotein, and other materials form. D. Plaque irritates tissue to form additional scar tissue and plaques, eventually blocking artery.

is cut off. The thickening process is known as *atherosclerosis* or hardening of the arteries. If an artery is closed off in the brain, the result is a stroke. If this happens to one of the vessels supplying the heart muscle, the result is a coronary or heart attack. Until relatively recently, it was thought that this process of plaque deposition did not begin until middle age. Now it is known that in our society the process has already begun in people who are in their late teens or early twenties.

OVERNUTRITION

Overnutrition and Obesity

Hunting-gathering man was typically in superb physical condition. Physical tone came about largely as a result of his dependence upon his own energy, rather than that of machines, to accomplish the day's tasks.

In contrast to hunting-gathering man, most of us are incredibly inactive. As Dr. Jean Mayer, a leading American nutritionist, has put it, the modern American ". . . man gets up, and, after briefly standing in front of his mirror using his electric toothbrush and his electric razor, sits down at the breakfast table, goes on to sit in his car, in his office, at coffee break, at lunch, in his office, in his car, at dinner, and in front of the television set; and, after lying in a warm bath for a while, goes on to lie in bed." [24]

In spite of his much greater physical activity, hunting-gathering man apparently ate less than we do. Some recent studies of Bushmen showed that they consumed about 2100 calories per day, compared to our excess of 3000. As a result of our ample diet, rich in fats and sugars, and our drastic reduction in physical activity, we face a health problem

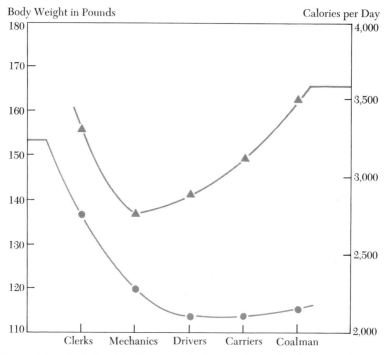

Figure 14-4. Relationship between body weight and caloric intake under various work situations. Five classes of Indian workers were studied by the American nutritionist, Dr. Jean Mayer. Although those in occupations involving much physical activity took in more calories than those in more sedentary occupations, they weighed less. (Data from Mayer, Jean, *Overweight*, Englewood Cliffs, New Jersey: Prentice-Hall, 1968.)

never before encountered; we are overweight. Until relatively recently, only the wealthy could afford the rich diet and the life of ease which leads to corpulence; at one time being fat was not something to be ashamed of, but was a mark of status.

The overweight person does not always eat more than others. Rather, the key to obesity lies in a loss of balance between caloric intake and energy expenditure. This is clearly shown by an interesting study which Dr. Mayer did among different groups of Indian workers. The work of these groups ranged from physically demanding to inactive. Although those engaged in heavy work ate more than those in sedentary occupations, the latter weighed more (Figure 14-4). In the same vein, anyone who has had a breakfast with lumberjacks or farm laborers knows that men in active physical work often consume great amounts of food, yet are less likely to be overweight than the city clerk who eats much less.

Obesity and Disease

Many insurance studies show that overweight people die earlier than others. Obesity leads to a greater likelihood of diabetes, kidney failure, and cardiovascular disease. Some studies seem to suggest that moderate obesity alone is not too critical a factor in causing heart attacks. When, however, it is combined with a high blood cholesterol level, the unlucky individual has a far higher chance of having arterial disease than if he had high cholesterol alone.

THE HUMAN MONOCULTURE

The Rise of the Human Monoculture

Primitive man was still a member of natural ecosystems. His technology was too weak to rework nature; thus he moved about in small, isolated bands, hunting and gathering. With the invention of agriculture, all this changed. The cultural ecosystems of agricultural man provided him with a new source of energy and at the same time, led him toward a new life style. Agricultural man removed himself from natural ecosystems and came to live in a man-made environment, first in villages, later in cities.

In several important respects, man's new environment resembled that of his domestic plants and animals. To illustrate this, one might think of the ways in which a wheat field resembles a city. First of all, both are monocultures, consisting of one major species, plus a few others, who are minor members of the monoculture. Second, both wheat field and city consist of dense aggregates of individuals. Third, both must continually fight off unwanted invaders. As you remember from Chapter 11, a cultural ecosystem such as a wheat field is constantly under attack from outsiders who would, if given a chance, move it back toward a stable condition of variety and complexity. Unfortunately, the same thing is true of a city. A variety of infectious organisms have followed man into his villages and cities, in effect attempting to reduce these simplified monocultural environments to a more normal state of complexity.

As the human monoculture has evolved, new and different infectious organisms have entered to exploit it. This process, which began with agricultural man, still continues today. In a way, a kind of

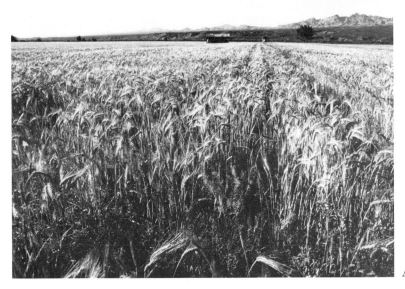

A.

Figure 14-5. The human monoculture: A. A wheat field in Arizona. (Courtesy of the U.S. Environmental Protection Agency.) B. A midwest suburb. (Chicago Aerial Survey.)

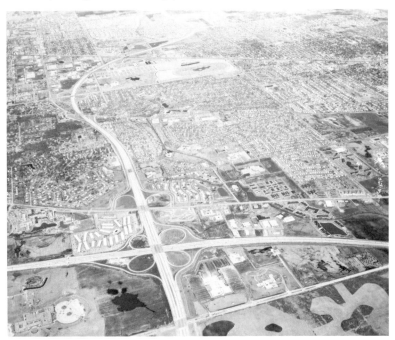

B.

sparring match continually takes place between man and organism. Sometimes we let our guard down by changing some aspect of our monoculture; this opens new pathways for infectious organisms to exploit. Sometimes the organisms themselves change. A mutant strain with a newly gained ability to survive in our environment will appear suddenly and may create an epidemic until we can devise new ways to seal it out of our monoculture. An infectious organism which has become newly established in our population is likely to be harder on its hosts than one which has been long established. For example, when venereal syphilis first became established in Europe, its effects were much more severe than is true for modern syphilis. The reduction in severity which takes place probably is largely the result of natural selection for compatibility (which is an advantage for both infectious organism and host).

What sorts of invaders are we locked in battle with today? Here are a few:

1. *Salmonellosis.* One of the biggest public health concerns in recent years has been the *Salmonella* problem. Salmonellosis is a kind of mild version of typhoid fever, with headache, chills, vomiting, and diarrhea. *Salmonella,* the group of bacteria causing this particular kind of food poisoning, has utilized several characteristics of Western technology to spread itself from host to host. In our affluent society we eat out much more often than ever before, often partaking of exotic foods which have been packaged under unsanitary conditions. In this way, we provide a convenient route for *Salmonella* to spread from non-Western cultures into our supposedly sanitary environment.

Salmonella commonly infects domestic fowl or their products. Since our food industry is highly mechanized, the *Salmonella* in one batch of infected eggs can be spread easily via mass mixing and mass distribution into many different cake-mix boxes or similar commercial products.

Salmonella also has taken advantage of a relatively recent pet fad. The small turtles one can buy in dime stores are commonly infected with *Salmonella.* Young children will play with infected turtles, then put their fingers in their mouths, thus creating another route for the bacterium to exploit.

2. *Farmer's lung.* Farmer's lung is an infectious disease perhaps as old as agriculture itself. The disease is caused by spores of a mold, *Microplyspora faeni,* which lives in moist hay. Breathing in the spores can cause chills, shortness of breath, and sometimes flulike symptoms. Farmer's lung is not an infection in the usual sense of the term, but

more of an allergy. Once exposed, a victim develops a sensitivity to the spore so that a reaction takes place whenever the spore is inhaled. One would expect that modern urban man would have escaped farmer's lung, but *M. faeni* has managed to move into our contemporary urban environment, taking advantage of our widespread use of air humidifiers. Increasing numbers of homes, office buildings, and even factories have installed air humidification systems. The damp evaporation pads or filters in humidification units are ideal breeding sites for the spore, which can then become airborne, infecting any residents or workers in the building. If you develop flulike symptoms a few hours after entering a building and lose them after leaving it, farmer's lung may be your problem. Other than staying away, or changing the system itself, little can be done. Disinfectants do not seem to prevent *M. faeni* from breeding.

3. *Hepatitis.* The virus causing *infectious hepatitis* probably has been with man for thousands of years. Largely disseminated through contaminated food and water, it causes fever, abdominal pain, and

THE EVOLUTION OF INFECTIOUS DISEASE

What kinds of infectious diseases did agricultural man have? We can only conjecture, but it seems probable that this new way of living provided openings for new kinds of infectious organisms that had been unknown to hunting-gathering man. For example, animal diseases such as anthrax and tuberculosis could now become established in man because they could be transmitted to him via village products such as milk, the skins of domestic animals, or even through the dust raised by domestic herds.

Agricultural village life created openings for new organisms to enter the human population in other ways. It has been suggested that the clearing of the forest in West Africa for agriculture may have marked the beginning of malaria. The organism which causes West African malaria is transmitted from host to host by mosquitoes which normally feed on great apes. Clearing the forest drove away the great apes and created new breeding sites for mosquitoes. The latter then turned to man for their meals.

As settled villages grew to preindustrial and finally industrial cities, a whole new spectrum of infectious diseases appeared. Some of these, such as cholera and typhoid fever, were water-borne and took ad-

jaundice or loss of liver function. Sometimes cases are mild, lasting only a few days. Other times they can be severe, lasting for months.

Serum hepatitis has approximately the same symptoms, but seems to be caused by a close relative, possibly a mutant strain, of the infectious hepatitis virus. This new virus seems to have taken advantage of two new routes of transmission from host to host—the drug needle and blood transfusions. Since the drug addict does not typically report his habit, public health officials have no way of making a direct survey of incidence. A few years ago serum hepatitis was increasing rapidly, presumably due to drug use. Now it has leveled off or even decreased as drug users take routes other than the needle. Blood transfusions, however, remain a major source of transmission. Drug addicts in need of money often become donors to commercial blood banks, and unfortunately it is not possible to check donated blood for the virus. Other potential routes for serum hepatitis may be ear piercing or tattooing the body.

4. *Influenza.* As is true for all of their kind, flu viruses can reproduce

vantage of the increasing lack of sanitation which accompanied the crowded conditions of life in these cities. Another group of infectious diseases, the contagions, were spread primarily from mouth to mouth via sneezing or coughing. Still others, particularly typhus and plague, were spread by the vermin which infested man's environment. Some of the infectious diseases, such as influenza, smallpox, and measles, are commonly self-limiting. That is, once having had the disease, a victim becomes immune to further attack for periods ranging from several months to a lifetime. Cities had to reach a certain size before they could support these new viruses—a size such that new uninfected persons would always be present to sustain the infection. Measles, for example, needs a host population of at least 300,000 to sustain itself.

Until very recently the infectious diseases have played a tremendously important role in history. Epidemics did more to win wars than battles ever did, and the great plague epidemics of Europe completely altered its economic structure.

Hans Zinsser's *Rats, Lice and History,* which is cited in the bibliography, is a fascinating study of the role typhus has played in the history of Europe.

only in a living cell. The viruses do this by invading our respiratory tract and attaching themselves to cells into which they empty their genetic materials. Once within the cell, these genes then command the infected cell to manufacture new virus particles. These then break out to repeat the cycle. From the flu virus' point of view, an ideal host is sick enough to sneeze and thus send out virus particles to new hosts but not sick enough to be isolated or to die, for either of these events means an end of the line for the resident viruses.

After being infected by a flu virus, we develop antibodies, which are proteins structured to defend us against further attack. In this way, an infected population will come to be immune against a particular strain of flu virus. Immunity can also be acquired artificially through vaccines, which are laboratory-grown, detoxified flu viruses. When injected, they produce mild cases of flu but still stimulate the body to produce antibodies against the real thing.

Unfortunately, the flu virus has a way of getting around these threats to its survival. Among the billions of viruses infecting a population, some will develop a fortuitous mutation—a structural change which allows them to penetrate the antibody barrier. These new mutant strains multiply rapidly and replace the old strain. Sometimes mutant forms are similar enough to old strains so that vaccines are still somewhat effective. But at roughly ten-year intervals, greatly altered strains suddenly appear, against which we have little or no defense. These

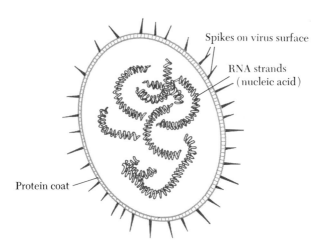

Spikes on virus surface

RNA strands
(nucleic acid)

Protein coat

Figure 14-6. The influenza virus. In some viruses, the nucleic acid or hereditary material is composed of RNA or ribonucleic acid rather than the DNA or deoxyribonucleic acid found in man.

cause the pandemics, the global flu epidemics. The greatest of these epidemics killed around twenty million people in 1918. Flu pandemics are still not understood. It may be that they are caused by hybrid strains of flu virus which have developed in some domestic animal. Suspicion centers on Chinese pigs since these animals are known to harbor flu viruses, and all pandemics, such as the Hong Kong flu of 1968–1969, seem to originate in the Orient.

5. *Shigella, and multiple drug resistance.* When the sulfa drugs and other antibiotics were first developed, many doctors hoped the answer to infectious disease had been found at last. Very soon, however, resistance strains appeared. The microorganisms causing staph infection, typhoid fever, venereal diseases, and many other infections have produced mutant strains which are increasingly resistant to different drugs, and doctors must either prescribe larger and larger doses of a given drug or use a battery of different drugs in an attempt to outwit the offending microorganisms.

Several years ago a new and ominous kind of drug resistance was discovered. The story begins with a drug-resistant strain of *Shigella,* the bacterium causing dysentery. This strain differed from others before it in the fact that it was resistant to *four* different drugs— sulfamilamide, streptomycin, chloramphenicol, and tetracyceline. Other strains of *Shigella* were soon found to also have multiple resistance to drugs. It was difficult to see how this could have happened through the usual process of mutation and natural selection, for the strains showing multiple resistance had appeared in patients who had received only one kind of drug. After a series of investigations it appeared that multiple drug resistance had appeared not through mutation alone but through a mutation combined with a kind of learning process. A large number of bacteria—some harmful, some not—reside in our intestines. In addition to the DNA carried within their nuclei, these bacteria also carry DNA in their plasmids, which are tiny particles outside the nucleus. During their life, bacteria of different kinds sometimes come together in *conjugation,* at which time they exchange their plasmids, and therefore they also exchange the genetic information contained in the DNA within the plasmids. Should the plasmids of some bacterium carry DNA which has mutated to produce resistance to a drug, this new mutant will be passed laterally to other kinds of bacteria through conjugation. For the bacteria this is a faster and more efficient way of spreading drug resistance—a number of different strains can pool their capacities and share their mutations for resistance.

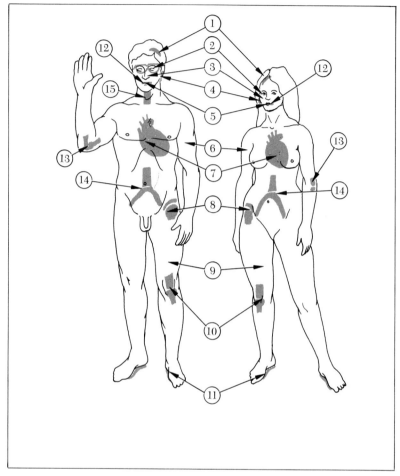

1. Skull plates
2. Glasses, contact lenses, corneal transplants
3. Plastic surgery
4. Hearing aids
5. False teeth
6. Vaccinations
7. Pacemaker, heart valves
8. Hip joints
9. Prosthetic devices
10. Knee joints
11. Arch supports
12. Pills, vitamins, etc.
13. Elbow joints
14. Dacron arteries
15. Speech-assistance devices

Figure 14-7. Some technological shields.

THE TECHNOLOGICAL SHIELD

Our technological environment may be creating still another health problem. In any other species beside man, natural selection acts as a kind of vast sieve which eliminates all but those organisms which are genetically best endowed to cope with the demands of their environment. Taken as a group, those who fail to reproduce are individuals who carry genes rendering them less able to cope with the environment than their peers. The cultural environment built by modern man interdicts this process of selection, for it provides a technological shield, a means of support which compensates for many genetic defects. Figure 14-7 shows some of the ways in which Western technology has compensated for genetic weaknesses. At earlier periods in man's history, those who carried defects such as these would have been at a selective disadvantage. Now, through the power of Western medical technology, they have been made as fit as others. Unfortunately, this may mean that in the long run our population will become burdened with an increasing frequency of bad genes. The dispute over whether this will happen leads to a larger dispute as to whether it is possible to speak about "good" or "bad" genes in any meaningful way.

Our technological shield acts in still another way to create a health problem. Since one of the shield's major effects is to preserve life, our average longevity is much greater than at any other time in history (Figure 13-6). This acts to increase the frequency of organic diseases such as cancer and heart attack for, in part, diseases such as these arise from the inevitable systemic failures that accompany the wear and tear of age.

15
TECHNOLOGICAL SOLUTIONS TO OUR HEALTH PROBLEMS

A number of technologies are being used or experimented with in the battle to reduce the health problems of our time. As we did in the case of environmental problems, we will not try to present an exhaustive review of these, but instead cite a few selected examples to give an idea of the kind of work being done.

CANCER

The Cause of Cancer

The greatest obstacle to the control of cancer is our ignorance of its true nature. Even though the cause of cancer is not yet understood, we do know a great deal about the ways in which cancer cells differ from normal cells. Three of these are of particular importance. First, cancer cells divide much more rapidly than do normal cells. Second, cancer cells have lost what biologists call *contact inhibition.* Normal cells will stop growing after contact with their neighbors. In contrast, cancer cells will keep on dividing. Third, cancer cells have lost the ability to recognize their own kind. If normal cells of several different tissues are mixed together in a laboratory preparation, they tend to sort themselves out. Cancer cells have lost this ability. Because of these traits, cancer cells form tumors, or masses of cells which continue to divide and spread until they kill their host.

Because the abnormal behavior of cancer cells is passed from generation to generation, it must somehow involve the cell's genetic material. How a cell's genetic machinery becomes altered to make it cancerous is the central problem of cancer research.

One theory holds that toxic substances in the environment cause a cell to mutate and become cancerous. The fact that many substances do have a carcinogenic action tends to support this idea. Another theory maintains that cancer is really a kind of infection. According to this view, the causative agent is a virus. Some biologists think a cancer-inducing virus infected mankind millions of years ago and is now a hidden part of our genetic machinery. Given the proper stimulus, these hidden viruses begin to reproduce, spreading from cell to cell and causing their host cells to become cancerous. Others maintain that cancer-causing viruses are more recent in origin and are passed to a victim either during his lifetime or perhaps from his mother before birth.

Great efforts have been made to identify viruses as the culprit in

PERSISTERS

When an epidemic of cholera rages through India, hundreds of thousands are stricken, yet most of the population seems to escape. Tests show that *subclinical infections,* in which a person carries the cholera bacterium but shows no sign of infection, are common. This pattern is found in many other infectious diseases and greatly complicates attempts at control, for in effect it is a mechanism by which potentially dangerous bacteria can hide themselves from detection. In some cases the microorganism can remain in an inactive state for years, then suddenly become active. In other cases a carrier who shows no symptoms of the disease may spread bacteria about the environment to infect others.

Viruses have evolved even more subtle and exasperating ways of hiding themselves than have bacteria. Tests can be made which show that potentially dangerous viruses are present in the body in some form, as *persisters,* although they cannot be identified by ordinary laboratory procedures. Since viruses multiply by inserting their genetic material into the host's cells and instructing the cells to build more viruses, it seems probable that viruses can commonly exist in a latent form by simply incorporating themselves into the host's genetic material and

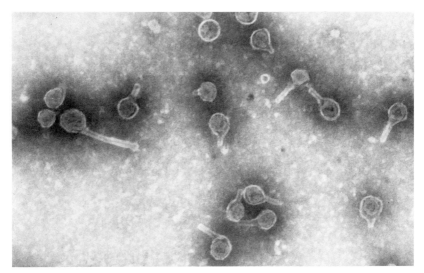

Figure 15-1. Rauscher leukemia viruses cause a mouse cancer. Magnification is 90,000 x. (Courtesy of Pfizer Inc.)

remaining there until some stimulus causes them to become active again. This ability of viruses to persist undetected in tissues has led to some unforeseen problems in vaccination technology. Most virus vaccines are made up of killed or inactive viruses of the disease in question. These produce minor disease symptoms and stimulate production of antibodies, which will then protect the body against future exposure to the live viruses of a real infection. One danger with virus vaccines is the possibility that other latent viruses might be injected along with the desired virus material. This apparently happened in the case of early lots of polio vaccine. These lots contained a hidden virus of a type later identified as SV (for simian virus) -40. SV-40 is a virus normally found in monkeys. When the first lots of polio vaccine were prepared, rhesus monkey tissue was used as the growth medium. This tissue apparently contained SV-40, and the virus was inadvertently introduced into people along with the polio vaccine.

There is some evidence that under some conditions, at least in hamsters, SV-40 can cause tumors; whether it may eventually become active and cause problems in those of us who presumably carry SV-40 is not known.

cancer. To date, the results have been mixed. Viruses have been found in association with animal tumors, and injection of these particles from one animal into another has produced new tumors. In man, some rather uncommon cancers, particularly one of African children called Burkitt's tumor, are known to be caused by a virus. Evidence is rapidly increasing that some sort of viruslike particle is associated with many other human cancers. Particles similar to the herpes virus, which causes cold sores, have been found in patients with Hodgkin's disease, a type of blood cancer, and in some cervical tumors. There is also some epidemiological evidence which suggests that cancers can be caught. Studies have been made which show that a number of people who have long known each other but are not related can sometimes come down with the same cancer. Actually, it is not surprising that it has proved so difficult to identify cancer viruses, for viruses have many ways of escaping detection. Until we have a thorough scientific understanding of cancer, however, we will be hampered in developing a really effective technology to treat it.

Treating Cancer

1. *Surgery.* Surgery is the treatment of choice for many cancers, and new techniques are being developed continually. A good example is some recent work by Dr. Robert Rand, a neurosurgeon at UCLA. Rand injects liquid silicone containing tiny iron spheres into a blood vessel near a tumor he wishes to treat. When the silicone reaches the tumor, a strong magnet is turned on, which holds the iron spheres and

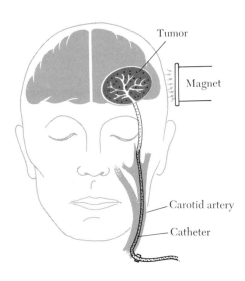

Figure 15-2. Method developed by Dr. Robert Rand for starving tumors. Catheter is threaded into carotid artery, and liquid silicone containing tiny iron spheres is pumped into tumor. Magnet holds silicone and iron in tumor while silicone hardens, blocking tumor's blood supply and thus killing it.

Figure 15-3.
Thermography is a technique in which heat-detecting devices can measure the heat radiated by tissues. Since tumors have a higher than average temperature, they can be located by this technique. Arrows indicate region of tumor. (Courtesy of the American Cancer Society.)

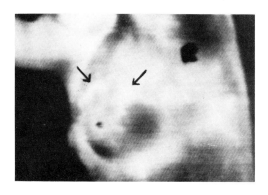

the silicone in place until the silicone hardens. This blocks the tumor's blood supply and kills it. The technique is limited to tumors with an easily isolated blood supply, and only a few operations have been done to date, but the results have been very promising.

One of the most damaging aspects of cancer surgery is its psychological impact. Breast cancer, for example, is normally treated by a radical mastectomy, in which the breast and surrounding tissue is removed. Although the psychological impact is often very severe, doctors have little choice. Even with treatment, breast cancer exacts a great toll— 71,000 women had breast cancer in 1971, and 30,000 of those were destined to die from it. Recently, the need for radical mastectomy has undergone a reexamination. Some studies suggest that a simple removal of the tumor is just as effective, at least in cases which are not too far advanced. For those who undergo a radical, plastic surgery with silicone implants has been a psychological aid. In either case, surgery is obviously a stop-gap therapy which hopefully will be replaced by drugs, immunization, or other more desirable treatments once we have a deeper understanding of the disease.

2. *Drugs.* A variety of drugs is used against cancer. Many current cancer drugs are antimetabolites, that is, they act to block cancer cells from gaining the nutritive materials they must have to keep growing. Some drugs whose development is based on the assumption that cancer is indeed caused by a virus are being tested. Dr. Richard Adamson of the National Cancer Institute has synthesized a drug, hydroxyguanidine, which attacks cancers in two ways. One part of the drug's molecule is tailored to interfere with the multiplication of cancer cells. Another part is derived from the guanidine molecule, which is known to interfere with the multiplication of viruses. To date, he has found his double-header drug to be effective in combating some animal cancers, and further tests are expected.

3. *Detection.* Attempts are being made to develop ways to detect cancer at a stage when it can be treated successfully. Some progress has been made toward this goal. A protein called carcinoembryonic antigen, or CEA, has been found to act as a kind of cancer indicator. Those with active cancers have larger amounts of CEA in their bodies than do normal persons. Recent work has shown that people who are destined to have cancer tend to have intermediate amounts of CEA— more than normal people, less than those with detectable cancers. CEA thus seems of potential value as a kind of early-warning signal for at least some kinds of cancer.

CARDIOVASCULAR DISEASE

Cardiovascular diseases are the leading cause of death in America today. Heart attacks alone strike a million Americans a year, nearly 700,000 of them fatally.

Many technologies are employed in the fight to control cardiovascular disease. Some of these involve radical strategies such as corrective or

BETTER LIVING THROUGH LESS TECHNOLOGY:

1. CARCINOGENS

In theory, one way to combat cancer would be to eliminate those things in our environment which seem to activate it. Various products of our technology, such as food additives or certain elements in air pollution, could be identified and then eliminated. Unfortunately, the list of material things which seem to induce cancer is almost endless.

Blacks in this country have less lip cancer than do whites, which seems due to the fact that fewer smoke pipes. On the other hand, esophageal cancer is higher among ghetto blacks, a difference which has been linked with the cheaper alcoholic beverages they consume.

Food habits are of importance. Icelanders have a high rate of stomach cancer, related, presumably, to a heavy diet of smoked fish. Japanese also have a high rate of stomach cancer. Here, both dietary and genetic factors may be involved.

Sometimes particular working conditions or kinds of behavior may lead to cancer. In the early part of this century, radium dial workers

transplant surgery. Others are aimed at managing cardiovascular disease through the use of medication or intensive care. Still others are designed to prevent the disease from appearing in the first place.

Radical Technologies

1. *Heart surgery.* Many heart attacks are caused by atherosclerosis in the coronary arteries. The coronaries are three rather small arteries which supply the heart muscle with blood. When their circulation is blocked, a portion of the heart muscle is killed, and the victim suffers a *coronary.* Coronary bypass operations, designed to correct this arterial failure, are now becoming common. A healthy blood vessel is implanted onto the heart as a substitute for the damaged coronary artery. Many other repair techniques are available, such as those to replace damaged valves or correct perforated septa within the heart.

2. *Surgery for stroke.* Every year a half million Americans are crippled by stroke. The paralysis which results from a stroke is often of a spastic type, in which the limbs are left twisted and helpless. In some way, a small region of the brain called the *pulvinar* seems to be

painted watch hands with luminous radium salts. This was done with a small paintbrush. From time to time, the workers would straighten the brush by placing it in their mouths. Only after it was too late was it realized that this practice led to cancer of the mouth.

Cervical cancer is strongly correlated with early sexual intercourse. It is more common among women who have had multiple partners and whose partners have not been circumcised. The more children a woman has, the more likely she is to have this sort of cancer. On the other hand, the likelihood of breast cancer decreases as a woman has an increasing number of children. Nursing one's children also lowers the likelihood of breast cancer.

Obviously, continued efforts will be made to identify and eliminate all those factors which predispose a person to cancer, but as one observer put it, in order to do this successfully it may be necessary to abolish the habit of living.

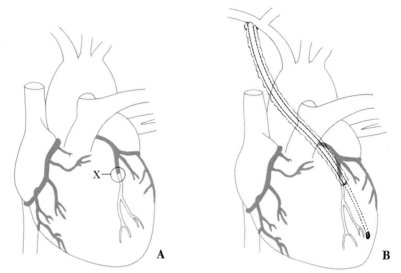

Figure 15-4. Coronary bypass. A. X marks a narrowing of the left coronary artery, causing a deficit in the blood supply to the heart. B. A coronary bypass, or implantation of a blood vessel to take the place of the artery and supply blood to the heart muscle.

associated with this paralysis. Using a tiny probe filled with liquid nitrogen, surgeons now can freeze some of the pulvinar's cells, which helps to relax the victim's affected limbs.

3. *Organ replacement.* Of all the surgical technologies directed toward the management of cardiovascular disease, the most spectacular is organ replacement. One school of thought maintains that we ought to concentrate our efforts in this area toward constructing a workable artificial heart. Artificial hearts have been implanted in animals with fair success, but many problems remain to be solved. For one thing, blood tends to clot on the surfaces of an artificial heart. For another the pumping action of an artificial heart can create areas of internal pressure which will damage blood cells. Also, since artificial hearts are not as efficient as real ones, they must be larger to do the work required of them.

Because of problems such as these, many medical scientists believe that implants of natural hearts hold more promise. However, if heart implantation is to become routine, the problem of transplant rejection must first be solved.

Homographs, or tissue transplants from one part of the body to another, are common operations in the field of plastic surgery. If you are an identical twin, you can also receive grafts from your other half with little trouble. In both of these situations, the grafted tissue has the same proteins or *antigens* as does the tissue of the recipient. In contrast, if you receive a graft from some unrelated person, it will contain antigens which your body recognizes as foreign. An implant of this type will activate your immune-response system. Certain cells in your blood and lymph systems will produce antibodies which act to fight off the invading tissue by attacking and neutralizing its antigens. The result will be localized inflammation and an eventual sloughing off or rejection of the graft. If this problem could be overcome, hearts and other kinds of organs could be transplanted routinely. In addition to living donors, organs could be taken from cadavers, or even, as has been suggested, from baboons and other primate donors, although these may be too small for effective use in man. At present, the immune reaction can be suppressed through drugs or radiation, both of which neutralize the lymphocyte cells which produce antibodies against a foreign graft. Unfortunately, the treatment neutralizes all lymphocytes,

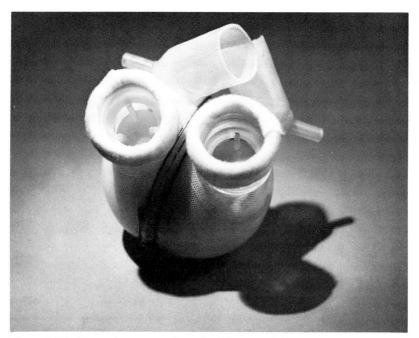

Figure 15-5. Kwan-Gett type of artificial heart. Fluffy circular openings are Dacron cuffs which would be sewed onto remnants of patient's atria. Ventricles are at bottom, aorta and pulmonary artery at upper right. Heart is designed to be driven by compressed air fed from outside patient. (Courtesy of Dr. W. J. Kolff, University of Utah.)

both those causing rejection and others which serve to protect the body against infective microorganisms. Thus, the price of a successful transplant is an extreme susceptibility to pneumonia or other infectious diseases.

The need, then, is to find some way to eliminate only those lymphocytes which act against the antigens of an implant, sparing the other lymphocytes which are needed to defend the body against infectious disease. Some promising progress has recently been made in this search. A group of medical researchers at the University of South Carolina have experimented with a closed-circuit system which removed lymph from cows. Glass beads, coated with an antigen foreign to the cow, were placed in the system (Figure 15-6). As the cow's lymphocytes flowed over the beads, those lymphocytes which were sensitive to the foreign antigen coated on the beads were removed from circulation. The researchers envision a similar system for human patients. The antigens of a prospective implant would be placed on the beads and the patient's lymph allowed to flow through the system. In this way, his blood would be cleansed of those particular lympho-

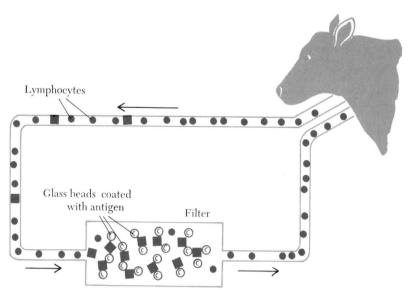

Figure 15-6. Closed-circuit filter system used experimentally with cows. Filter contains antigen. The cow's lymph, a fluid which forms part of the circulatory system, flows through the filter. Those lymphocytes (square shapes) which are sensitive to the antigen are removed; other lymphocytes (circles) pass back to cow's circulation.

cytes which would reject the graft, but other kinds would not be affected.

Dr. William Summerlin of New York's Sloan-Kettering Institute has found that skin grafts are less prone to be rejected if they are kept for a time in the kind of nutrient solution used to culture cells. He has been able to successfully implant the skin of a pig treated in this way onto mice. The technique is being further investigated with the possibility in mind that it might be used in human grafts.

Much basic research also is being directed toward gaining a better understanding of the immune response itself. Recently it has been found that there are really two immune systems. B lymphocyte cells are programmed to ward off a variety of infectious bacteria. T cells, a second sort of lymphocyte, react against viruses and the antigens of grafts. The genetics of the system is also being worked out. As of now, four pairs of genes have been identified which control the immune system in man.

4. *Regeneration.* Many lower animals can regenerate lost or damaged parts. In man and most other higher species, this ability has been lost. If we knew enough about the biology of regeneration, it might be possible to turn the process on artificially in order to regrow damaged hearts or other organs. Recently Robert Becker, a professor of orthopedic surgery at the State University of New York, has made progress in this direction. He inserted tiny electrodes into the stumps of severed limbs of rats. A very low level of electric current was then introduced. Becker's rats have responded by regenerating portions of their limbs, and he is now trying the technique on human bone fractures where regrowth has been incomplete.

Management Technologies

1. *Drug therapy.* At least thirty million Americans have high blood pressure, and the actual figure is probably far higher. Normally, the pressure in our blood vessels is regulated through a complex control system of hormones, other chemicals, and nerves. Under some conditions, the control system goes awry and sends disruptive signals which cause an excessive constriction of the vessels, resulting in dangerously high blood pressure. Various drugs have been developed to try to manage high blood pressure. Certain nitrate compounds do this, apparently by controlling the abnormal signals. Other drugs tranquilize the patient and are used on the assumption that the basic cause for hypertension is our stressful life style.

Drugs are also used to treat heart disease. Nitroglycerin is still the medication of choice to ward off angina, the intense pain that is associated with a failure of a diseased coronary artery to feed the heart adequately.

2. *Supportive care.* Respiratory failure sometimes follows major surgery such as that involving the heart. It may also be associated with organic failures such as heart attack or emphysema. In respiratory failure, the small air sacs or *alveoli* of the lungs are no longer able to take oxygen from the capillaries surrounding them. This may be due to their collapse or to an obstruction within them. As a result, the oxygen level in the bloodstream falls, which in turn affects the entire metabolism of the body. When this happens the patient may be placed in an intensive care unit where his respiratory system will be supported and controlled artificially until it can reestablish itself. A

BETTER LIVING THROUGH LESS TECHNOLOGY:

2. STRESS

In theory, one way to reduce cardiovascular disease would be to ease the stress in our society. The city is certainly our most stressful environment. Here, for example, is the way New York impressed one newcomer.

"When I first came to New York it seemed like a nightmare. As soon as I got off the train at Grand Central I was caught up in pushing, shoving crowds on 42nd Street. Sometimes people bumped into me without apology; what really frightened me was to see two people literally engaged in combat for possession of a cab. Why were they so rushed? Even drunks on the street were bypassed without a glance. People didn't seem to care about each other at all." [25]

Many of us have experienced the same sort of emotions, yet if we have spent any amount of time in a large city, we soon learn to adjust. How do we go about doing this? Stanley Milgram has made a study of the way urbanites adapt to the stress of city life. He finds that, unlike country people, city dwellers have developed behavior patterns which enable them to selectively shut out some aspects of the urban environment. Here are some of these patterns:

1. Although he is in contact with hundreds of individuals every day,

tube is passed, either via the mouth or by incision below the Adam's apple, into the patient's lungs, so that gas can be introduced directly from a ventilator. The oxygen content of the gas can be adapted to compensate for the degree of failure in the patient's lungs. Since the oxygen-absorbing ability of the patient's lungs will vary, his state is monitored constantly by checking the amount of carbon dioxide in his blood. Intensive metabolic management of this kind has proved highly successful, but it does submerge the patient within a rather bewildering array of medical technology.

Less complicated techniques are being developed which are also designed to support the patient's body until it can recover normal function. Sometimes a heart is so badly damaged that it cannot maintain adequate blood circulation in the body. Blood pressure falls, and the patient will die if the pressure is not restored to normal levels.

an urbanite has a personal relationship with only a few of these people. In a small town, everyone is likely to greet everyone else on the street. In a city, one makes little attempt to become acquainted with other pedestrians or the clerks in a department store.

2. This social anonymity extends to many crisis situations. City people tend to develop an indifference to the personal problems of others. As our observer noted, few pedestrians on a crowded city street will stop to help a drunk. Physical contacts are deliberately kept at an impersonal level. For example, two people bumping into each other often will not apologize.

3. A city dweller develops many filtering devices which reduce his contact with those about him. He often has an unlisted phone or will look through a peephole before deciding whether to answer the door.

Stress-reducing behavior of this kind raises some interesting questions. First, one might ask whether it is logical to build an environment and then try to shut out this environment. Second, one might ask if a city, with all of its potential for fulfilling human needs, must inevitably lead to stress overload or whether we could design a city with an acceptable stress level. Finally, one wonders if we might design an environment from which too much stress has been filtered.

A gadget called the *intra-aortic balloon pump assist* has been designed to help the heart while it regains normal strength. A deflated balloon is threaded into a leg vein and then up into the aorta, the body's largest artery. The balloon is then timed to inflate synchronously with the ailing heart, to give it a boost in its work of sending blood through the circulatory system.

Preventive Technologies

Some promising work is under way in the attempt to develop drugs which would act to prevent cardiovascular disease. A drug named clofibrate, which acts to lower the cholesterol level in blood, is being tested to see whether it will help to prevent heart attacks. In a five-year study, 700 United Airlines ground personnel took clofibrate, while another 700 were given a placebo, a pill identical in appearance but without the drug. Among older men in the untreated group, the heart-attack rate was three and a half times higher than in the treated group. Among younger men it was over eight times higher.

Some medical researchers think high bood pressure is caused more by an excess of sodium in the body than by stress or other environmental factors. Thus, drugs which release sodium from the body are being experimented with in an attempt to prevent hypertension.

BETTER LIVING THROUGH LESS TECHNOLOGY:

3. BIOFEEDBACK

As conceptualized by Western biology, the activities of our body are either under voluntary or involuntary control. Arm and eye movements, for example, are under voluntary control. In contrast, a heartbeat, a churning stomach, a blush, or the constriction of blood vessels associated with high blood pressure are under involuntary control. These latter activities are largely mediated by the autonomic nerve system but also by hormones.

Eastern meditation systems, notably Yoga and Zen Buddhism, have never accepted this dichotomy. Yogis, for example, long have claimed the ability to control their bodies' metabolism. Many accounts exist in which Yogis have regulated their heartbeat or have managed to survive long periods underground while in a kind of hibernation. At

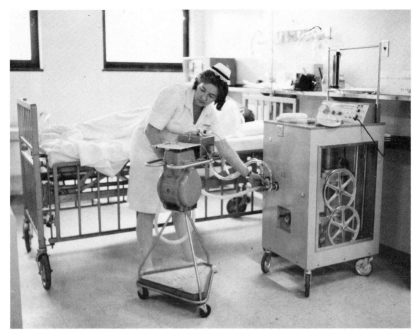

Figure 15-7. Respiratory therapist adjusts respirator in an Intensive Care Unit at Massachusetts General Hospital, Boston. (Courtesy of MGH News.)

first, Western science ignored these claims; now opinion is changing. A number of experiments have shown that through meditation it is indeed possible to control physiological behavior that formerly was thought to be involuntary. Meditation, for example, can cause a decline in blood lactate level, a rise in electrical resistance of the skin, and a change in alpha brain waves. In the last several years, increasing attention has been given to these so-called *biofeedback* techniques. Most interest has centered on the achievement of desired mental states, but increasingly those who are working in this area are turning toward the possibility of using biofeedback to restrain the body's involuntary reactions to stress stimuli and thus develop a new approach to the control of organic disease.

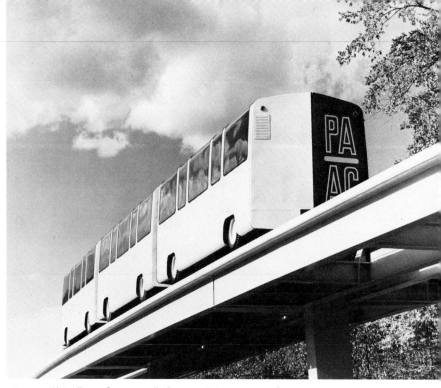

Figure 15-8. "People mover" designed by Westinghouse Corporation. Vehicle is electrically powered, runs on tires, and can be linked into "trains" as shown in this photograph. Transport systems such as this would drastically reduce the accident rate of automobile travel and would greatly help to reduce America's dependency on fossil fuel. (Courtesy of Westinghouse Corporation.)

ACCIDENTS

Many different technologies have been proposed in an attempt to lower the accident rate in the Western world. Many are concerned with the hazards of transport systems, particularly automobiles. One proposal, which would have the additional values of economy and efficiency, is the Electrocar system. The gasoline-powered car of today would be replaced by a uniformly designed vehicle, the Electrocar. Although Electrocars could be individually owned, many—perhaps most—would be leased as part of a centrally organized system. Much Electrocar travel would be on guideways, or central routes comparable to our present interstate and state highways. When on these guideways Electrocars would be locked into a central source of electrical power which would move them along at a fixed speed. Because of this, travel would be almost completely accident free. Any one guideway could handle ten times the traffic one of our present interstate lanes now handles. When off a guideway, Electrocars could be operated manually, drawing on battery power. The battery could be recharged during guideway travel or at night when the car is not in use. Of course, a system of this kind would mean some sacrifice of individuality.

Solutions such as these are ingenious, but they could only work if we realigned our values with respect to the real function of our technology. As industrial designer Victor Papanek has said,

> the automobile has become so overloaded with false values that it has emerged as a full-blown status symbol, dangerous rather than convenient. It breathes and exhales a great amount of cancer-inducing fumes, it is overly fast, wastes raw materials, is clumsy, and kills 50,000 people in an average year.[26]

Whether the American public would accept the regimentation implicit in an Electrocar system is an interesting point and raises issues we will return to in Part III of this book.

INFECTIOUS DISEASES

With the possible exception of cancer, the common cold and influenza are the last great infectious diseases of Western man.

At the present time, a number of research projects are under way in an attempt to build new and better vaccines against influenza. French scientists have claimed success in developing vaccines which anticipate new flu pandemics. These scientists say that they have been able to evolve a variety of mutant strains of flu and then to build vaccines against these strains. Whether the new vaccines will indeed anticipate those new strains of influenza virus which are bound to evolve over the next few years remains to be seen.

The common cold is a virus disease of great economic and nuisance importance, but an effective vaccine against it may soon be developed. A protein called interferon may play a key role in such a vaccine. Interferon, first discovered in the 1950's by English researchers, is produced by white blood cells in direct response to viral infections. Earlier attempts to use it as a vaccine failed, possibly because small doses were used. In more recent tests, heavy doses were given to half of 32 persons exposed to cold viruses. Of those receiving interferon, none had any cold symptoms, while thirteen of the sixteen controls caught cold. Interferon is a nonspecific protein, combating a variety of virus infections, and thus might be effective against other viruses in addition to those causing the common cold. At present it is too expensive for wide usage, as one dose costs several thousand dollars.

Some progress also is being made in developing a vaccine for serum hepatitis. In 1971 patients at Willowbrook State Hospital on Staten Island in New York were inoculated with inactivated serum from infected patients and then exposed to serum from patients who had the disease. A two-year follow-up study was made to see whether this treatment made the experimental subjects resistant to serum hepatitis. The data seem to indicate that this has happened.

GENETIC DISEASE

Over 1,600 human diseases are associated with some kind of hereditary defect. Although most of these are rare, some, such as sickle cell anemia, cystic fibrosis and mongolism, are not.

While no one really knows, many biologists feel that a number of these diseases are on the increase as a result of Western technology's ability to shield those with genetic disease from the action of natural selection. Concern about this coupled with a desire to eliminate genetic diseases and the anguish they can cause, has led to the development of several management technologies. Some of these are already under way; others are only proposed. Some are relatively mild programs; others are radical in the amount of control and change they advocate. All have a common aim: to eliminate deleterious genes in modern man.

Genetic Counseling

Sickle cell anemia is an hereditary disease in which the red blood cells carry abnormal hemoglobin molecules, which link together to form long, rigid chains. These force the normally disk-shaped blood cells into a sickled form. The abnormal cells tend to bunch together, clogging blood vessels. This causes great pain, anemia, and a variety of complications. Sickle cell disease is usually fatal and no really effective treatment is known. The genetics of the disease is relatively simple, for only two genes, S and s, are involved. A person with an SS genotype is normal; an ss genotype produces the disease. Ss people are called carriers. Under normal conditions, carriers show no symptoms of the disease. Two carriers, however, can have children with the disease. In the United States, the incidence of the s gene, and thus of sickle cell anemia, is much higher among blacks than among whites. The reason for this relates to conditions in tropical Africa, the ancestral home of most American blacks. Until recently, malaria was very common in Africa. It turns out that a person who has an Ss genotype has a greater resistance to malaria than does an SS individual. As a

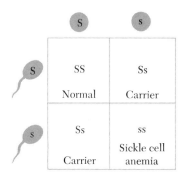

Figure 15-9. How two carriers can produce a child with sickle cell anemia. S or s sperm of man (left) can combine with S or s eggs of woman (top) to produce the four offspring shown in box. Thus, there is a one-fourth chance that any one of their offspring will be an ss and have the disease.

result, natural selection among black Africans favored those with the Ss genotype, which kept the frequency of the s gene at a high level. When black slaves first were brought to this country three hundred years ago, as many as one quarter carried the Ss genotype. Since there was no advantage in having the Ss genotype in America, natural selection operated against the s gene, and now only about ten per cent of American blacks have the Ss genotype.

Since several tests are available to show whether or not a person is a carrier, it is becoming possible for a couple contemplating marriage to be counseled as to the probability that they will have children with the disease. If two carriers marry, a 25 per cent chance exists that any one child will have sickle cell anemia, and there is a 50 per cent chance that a child will be a carrier (Figure 15-9).

In a number of other hereditary diseases, the genetics is also simple enough to allow a counselor to make qualified predictions. These diseases include cystic fibrosis, hemophilia, Huntington's chorea, and Tay-Sach's disease. In other genetic diseases such as Down's Syndrome, or mongolism, the situation is not as clear, but a counselor still can be of some aid. Through genetic counseling, it is possible to discourage those who have a high risk of producing defective children from doing so.

One problem with genetic counseling is the uncertainty which accompanies it. A counselor may advise a carrier of the sickle cell gene that he or she should avoid having children or at least be aware of the hazards involved, but there always remains a factor of uncertainty —all advice must be given in terms of probabilities.

Amniocentesis

A medical technology developed in the last few years may help to surmount some of the uncertainty associated with counseling. This

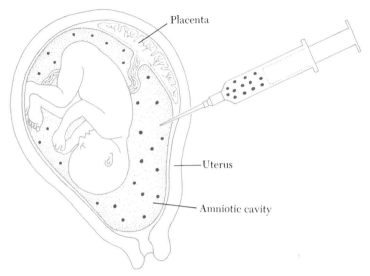

Figure 15-10. Amniocentesis. Fluid surrounding the fetus is withdrawn by a syringe. Both the amniotic fluid and loose cells from the fetus can then be tested for genetic abnormalities.

technique, called amniocentesis, examines the genetic makeup of an individual before he is born. The fluid which surrounds a developing fetus is filled with cells shed from the fetus' skin and respiratory tract. With relatively little danger to the mother or fetus, an experienced physician can insert a needle and withdraw some of this fluid. The fourth month of pregnancy seems to be the best time for this, as the fetus has not developed enough to be in the way, but enough fluid is available to make its collection relatively easy. Fetal cells are taken from the fluid and grown in tissue culture. Both the fluid and the cells are then examined in various ways for hereditary abnormalities. Over forty genetic diseases can be diagnosed by this method. The mother and her physician can thus be warned of trouble ahead and decide whether an abortion is desirable (Figure 15-10).

Muller's Scheme

H. J. Muller, the late Nobel laureate, was deeply concerned about the genetic deterioration he felt was taking place in modern society. His answer to the problem was to use the idealism and self-interest of individuals as a lever to improve our genetic stock. Many couples cannot have children because the husband either is sterile or, in some cases, has a genetic deficiency which makes reproduction inadvisable.

Sometimes such couples resort to AID, or artifical insemination by an anonymous donor, who is usually chosen by the couple's physician. Muller felt it would make more sense to use the sperm of someone whose characteristics were known. If sperm banks could be set up containing the sperm of men prominent in various fields, the couple could then choose those traits they wished for in their offspring. Muller felt that those who would pioneer this method would tend to be "idealistic, humanistic, and at the same time realistic persons, who will tend to have especially well-developed values." [27] These people would tend to seek traits such as intelligence or curiosity, and certainly they would avoid sperm which might carry genetic disease.

Since Muller first suggested his idea, sperm-bank technology has developed to the point where individuals can and do deposit sperm for use in the future. Up to now, those who have done so are men who have had vasectomies and are buying insurance—maintaining a supply of their sperm, should they later wish to father children. Sperm are kept in glycerine and stored in liquid nitrogen. Under an expanded system, the sperm from thousands of individuals, from great artists to athletes, could be stored for future use by couples wishing to blend a particular kind of genetic aptitude into their children.

Building a Perfect Man

Programs of the sort we have just described do not go far enough for some biologists. A more efficient way of creating a population of healthy individuals would be to design them from scratch, to build human beings who are perfectly adapted to their environment.

This sort of thinking sends shudders down most people's spines, but steps toward this end are already being taken.

1. *In vitro reproduction.* In order to produce made-to-order people, it would be necessary to mechanize the reproductive process. Over the last twenty years a number of experimenters have set the stage for this. Normally human ovaries produce only one egg per month. With hormones, it is now possible to induce ovaries to increase their egg production many times. Removing these eggs is then a relatively simple process. A surgeon simply inserts two tubes into the women's abdomen. One is equipped with a small light, the other with a suction tube. The removed eggs can then be placed in nutrient solutions and sperm added. Some eggs which have been fertilized and grown outside the womb or in vitro have developed to a fairly advanced embryonic stage. Work with animals suggests that artificial placentas and the other technologies needed for growth to term will be available

soon. When this happens, it would be possible to choose an ideal man and woman and produce hundreds of offspring from their gametes. In vitro reproduction may remind one of Huxley's classic anti-utopian novel *Brave New World,* but it is now a technology well past the science fiction stage, one close to being a reality. Other even more radical technologies loom.

2. *Cloning.* Suppose one takes a fertilized salamander egg and places a ligature around it so that the nucleus is confined to one half (Figure 15-11A). The half with the nucleus is then allowed to divide into sixteen cells (Figure 15-11B). If one of the nuclei from the sixteen cells is now allowed to escape into the left half and the halves are separated, each will form a normal adult salamander (Figure 15-11C). This indicates that at the sixteen-cell stage the nuclei are *totipotent,* that is, they have the ability to direct formation of a complete adult. If on the other hand the cells are allowed to divide to later stages and the experiment is repeated, the left half will form an abnormal adult. At later stages the nuclei have lost their totipotency, and each cell has become *determined,* or capable of forming only one kind of

EUGENICS

Eugenicists are biologists or others who fear that a generalized deterioration of our genetic stock is taking place. To many eugenicists, this *dysgenic* trend implies more than an increase in genetic disease. It also implies that the protective shield created by our technology acts to remove those who are socially unfit from the pressures of natural selection. The assumption is that genes (assuming that such exist) for traits such as laziness, low I.Q. and the like are therefore on the increase. Some eugenicists fear that our fast-paced, violent, over-organized society will eventually select genes so as to create a race of insensitive, thick skinned people who have no sense of individuality, who are completely subordinate to group interests.

Concerns such as these have led many eugenicists to advocate positive eugenics programs in which society would choose individuals with ideal genotypes and encourage these people to reproduce. The kind of encouragement suggested has ranged from financial rewards to strict state control of reproduction.

Positive eugenics programs are open to some very serious criticisms. For one thing, the whole area of human genetics is still so little known

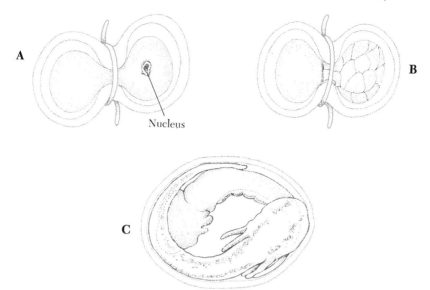

Figure 15-11. Experiment showing how a salamander nucleus retains its totipotency through the sixteen-cell stage. See text for explanation.

that most of the eugenicists' misgivings are based on conjecture rather than fact. We don't know just what genetic trends are taking place, and for that matter we don't know whether traits such as laziness or insensitivity have a genetic base, and if so, what their nature is.

Another objection is that we really cannot rate a genetic trait as "good" or "bad" in any absolute sense. As the text suggests, while it is bad to have the genotype Ss today, this was not so a hundred years ago in Africa. Similarly, while we might today judge togetherness as bad and individuality as good, our evaluation might be just the opposite when made in the context of our society a hundred years from now.

Still another objection has to do with the efficiency of selection procedures for desirable traits. All studies indicate that unless police-state methods are used, selection rates would be very slow, even if considerable social pressure were applied to encourage those people with more desirable characteristics to reproduce.

The greatest objection to positive eugenics programs is of course the moral one. Who will play God and decide who is to be favored?

tissue. If some way could be found to keep or to regain the characteristic of totipotency, it would be possible to take an adult salamander, divide it into its millions of component cells, and from each grow an identical replica of the original salamander. If we could discover the key to totipotence in any animal, we would be well on the way to repeating the process in man. In other words, we could create *clones,* or colonies of millions of identical people, all derived from the tissue of one parent. Some progress in this direction has been made. In other experiments, when the nucleus from an older determined frog cell was transferred to a newly fertilized egg from which the nucleus had been removed, this hybrid cell developed into a normal frog. Somehow its new surroundings changed the determined nucleus back toward a state of totipotency.

Even if man could be cloned, those who managed the production line would have relatively little control over the specific genetic makeup of their product. A third technology, gene insertion, might someday achieve this goal.

3. *Gene insertion.* Since viruses insert themselves into the genetic material of a cell, it should be possible to use a virus as a kind of messenger, allowing it to infect a cell with genetic material of one's choice. Work has just begun on gene insertion, but results to date suggest that it may prove to be a feasible tactic. If so, the way would be open to build cells which meet certain genetic specifications and to develop human clones from these.

What characteristics might an ideal production line individual have? Here are a few suggestions: self cleansing arteries built to ward off atherosclerosis; a stress system that is tuned to the stress of our civilization; an altered respiratory tract with built-in pollution detector and filter; and extra ventricle so that this particularly vulnerable part of the heart would have a spare; a digestive system geared to a fat- and sugar-laden diet; half-size individuals with a slower reproductive rate to hold down crowding and thus decrease the stress of life on this planet.

THE CONQUEST OF AGE

A large number of our health problems are age-related; they seem to crop up with increasing frequency as we move past middle and into old age. To some researchers, old age itself is just another disease which finally claims us, should we escape all others. To regain one's youth—perhaps even to become immortal—has always been a dream of man-

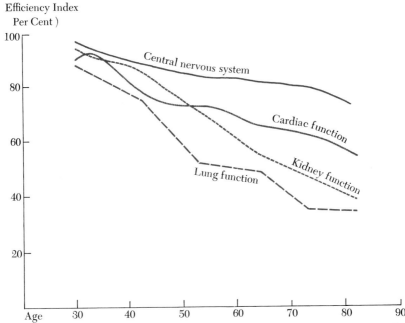

Efficiency Index
Per Cent)

Central nervous system

Cardiac function

Kidney function

Lung function

Age

Figure 15-12. Changes associated with aging. Central nervous system index is based on distance a nerve impulse travels in a second. Lung function index is volume of air inhaled and expelled in one minute. Cardiac function index is based on blood pumped per minute, kidney function index on blood flow through kidneys.

kind, but now some medical scientists see it as more than a dream. Many research teams are actively exploring the mystery of aging. Aging normally is thought of as a slowing of bodily functions. Eyesight and hearing fail, the breath shortens, and by a variety of measurements (Figure 15-12) one's body begins to fail. The vital question is: What causes this? Here are five hypotheses which have been suggested to account for aging:

1. The body's DNA is programmed to fail after a given period of time. This hypothesis receives support from work by Dr. Leonard Hayflick of Stanford University, who has demonstrated that human fibroblast cells give out after approximately fifty divisions. Hayflick's experiments have indicated that this failure is not due to accumulation of waste or exhaustion of nutrients or any other extrinsic factor; it seems to be built into the genetic code itself.

2. Cells age because their DNA slowly fails through *copy error*. As the DNA divides and moves into daughter cells, tiny mistakes take

place. Given enough time, these mistakes accumulate until the DNA strands of aged cells can no longer direct the cell's activity adequately.

3. Aging results from *cross linkage*. This is a tendency for large protein molecules to become entangled chemically, impeding cell metabolism.

4. Aging is due to auto-immune reactions. Over the years, the body's mechanism for manufacturing antibodies may become damaged through mutations in the DNA which directs antibody manufacture. As a result, the body's immune mechanism would no longer recognize some of the body's own tissue as friendly; it would identify it as foreign protein and manufacture antibodies against this tissue. Some diseases such as arthritis act as if they may be in part a result of such an immune reaction.

5. Aging is due to the accumulation of age pigments in the non-dividing cells of the body. These are largely located in the heart, brain, and muscles.

No one knows which if any of these hypotheses really accounts for aging. Even though the basic causes remain to be discovered, medical science is working to understand old age, after which appropriate technologies could be developed. Even before this understanding has been achieved, some crude technologies to combat aging are already being tried. Reducing body temperature seems to delay the aging process, as does a reduction of caloric intake. Various drugs are being experimented with. Some of these act to break up the cross linkage that many researchers feel is the key factor in aging. Other drugs work against the accumulation of age pigments.

Our technology has developed or proposed many solutions for Western man's health crisis. If these solutions are to work at all, we must ask those same questions we raised at the end of the chapter on technological solutions for our ecological crisis: Will more technology solve problems which were created by technology? Can we continue to expand our technological environment and still retain our human qualities?

We turn to these questions in Part III.

FUTURE

In Part II we have described modern Western technology as somewhat two-faced. It has brought us more power than mankind has ever before seen. With this power Western man has fashioned a material world of great complexity and sophistication. This technological environment holds the promise of liberating man from the traditional constraints of hard work, pain, and boredom which have always been his lot. On the other hand, this new environment has brought with it a special set of problems. Natural resources have been depleted, natural ecosystems disrupted. While traditional diseases have been all but eliminated, a new set of technological diseases have arisen to take their place.

In Part II we also described a number of technological fixes—ways in which technology might be employed to solve these problems. These were offered in an uncritical spirit, as if there were no question but that they would lead us away from our troubles. Questions, however, do exist. How do we know that more technology would not simply produce more trouble? Would it not be better to think in terms of unpacking some of our technology, moving back in time toward a simpler, more natural environment, closer to that under which we evolved? If we do decide to take the technological route, what particular dangers should we watch for?

In this last part of the book we will consider these questions.

16 _____UNKNOWNS

In Part II we spent considerable time discussing the causes of the problems which seem to stem from life in a technological environment. Before we begin our critical assessment of technological solutions, it may be wise to take a look at some areas of disagreement respecting these technological problems. In this way, we can begin with a better perspective, which means we will have a realization of how little we really know about the whole problem.

Three issues are of central concern to anyone who wishes to attack the problems created by Western technology.

1. How much control do we really have over the direction our technology will take?

2. How strongly is man's behavior bound to his biological past?

3. How serious is the technological crisis in the Western world?

HOW MUCH CONTROL DO WE REALLY HAVE OVER THE DIRECTION OUR TECHNOLOGY WILL TAKE?

On first reading, this probably seems an odd sort of question. This is so because most of us are "free-willers." We automatically assume we can shape the future, including our technology, in almost any fashion we wish, at least within the constraints of the natural environment.

225

A small but vocal school of *determinists*, however, argues that we delude ourselves. To the determinists, man has no free will; he is actually a kind of prisoner within his culture. To the determinists it is culture, and particularly technological culture, which molds man's actions and beliefs. Free-willers disagree. To them man has personal control over his beliefs and values. These determine his technology and thus his material environment. If man is dissatisfied with his environment, he need only to reshape his beliefs and values; his technology and material environment will then follow suit.

Two Free-Willers: Lynn White, Jr. and Theodore Roszak

In a now-classic paper titled "The Historical Roots of our Ecologic Crisis" the historian Lynn White, Jr. has built a persuasive argument that man's beliefs condition his technology. Before the advent of Christianity, Northern Europe was pagan. Just as do the Bushmen, early Europeans saw themselves as a part of the natural environment. Each rock, stream, or tree had its particular spirit. Before one took from nature, these spirits had to be placated. The pagan European lived in an intimate relationship with his surroundings. His world was an animistic one, peopled with centaurs, fauns, and mermaids. Christianity, however, destroyed this view and substituted a far different one. As White puts it, "Christianity, in absolute contrast to ancient paganism and Asia's religions (except, perhaps, Zoroastrianism), not only established a dualism of man and nature but also insisted that it is God's will that man exploit nature for his proper ends." [28] In the older paganism, the world had no visible beginning or end. In Christianity the idea of progress toward the goal of salvation became important. With this idea came the belief that man's proper role on earth was that of transforming it, rebuilding it in the image of God and man.

In the older paganism, man and other creatures existed together in an intimate relationship. Under Christianity the world exists solely for man.

> By gradual stages a loving and all-powerful God had created light and darkness, the heavenly bodies, the earth and all its plants, animals, birds, and fishes. Finally, God had created Adam and, as an afterthought, Eve to keep man from being lonely. Man named all the animals, thus establishing his dominance over them. God planned all of this explicitly for man's benefit and rule: no item in the physical creation had any purpose save to serve man's purposes. And, although man's body is made of clay, he is not simply part of nature: he is made in God's image. [29]

Thus, Christianity is one of the most egocentric religions the world has ever seen. In most religions, man is a part of nature, but under Christianity, nature exists to serve man. Dante's view of the universe (Figure 8-1A) again serves to illustrate this point.

Although, as White notes, many of us are not practicing Christians, our daily habits are dominated by this view of reality. Because of this, White argues that no amount of science or technology will solve the problems that flow from our alienation from nature. What is needed is a qualitatively different kind of world view. As a model for this new view of reality, White suggests a great Christian heretic: Saint Francis of Assisi. Founder of the Franciscan Order, Francis tried to counter Christian orthodoxy by removing man from his pedestal and making him an equal, not a superior among other species.

White concludes his paper this way:

> The greatest spiritual revolutionary in Western history, Saint Francis, proposed what he thought was an alternative Christian view of nature and man's relation to it: he tried to substitute the idea of the equality of all creatures, including man, for the idea of man's limitless rule of creation. He failed. Both our present science and our present technology are so tinctured with orthodox Christian arrogance toward nature that no solution for our ecologic crisis can be expected from them alone. Since the roots of our trouble are so largely religious, the remedy must also be essentially religious, whether we call it that or not. We must rethink and refeel our nature and destiny. The profoundly religious, but heretical, sense of the primitive Franciscans for the spiritual autonomy of all parts of nature may point a direction. I propose Francis as a patron saint for ecologists.[30]

Many others share White's view that our troubles stem not from technology per se, but from our view of the world. Theodore Roszak, for example, sees our problems in this way. Unlike White, however, Roszak's prime villain is not Christianity, but modern science. In his books *The Making of a Counter Culture* and *Where the Wasteland Ends* Roszak has developed a powerful case for the idea that science has in effect forced the West to look upon the world from its own particular viewpoint. Science has taught us that good is equated with reason and that to be emotional is somehow less desirable than to be detached and objective. Roszak's objection to this way of looking at the world is that it spawns a society in which individuals become alienated from each other and from the natural environment. Instead of bringing us toward a clearer vision of reality, Roszak thinks science has taken us toward an overly abstract, unreal picture of the world, one devoid of the emotions and feelings which are such a necessary part of being alive.

In *Where the Wasteland Ends* Roszak sums up his view thus: "My argument has been that single vision, the ruling sensibility of the scientific world view, has become the boundary condition of human consciousness within urban-industrial culture, the reigning Reality Principle, the whole meaning of sanity." Does this mean that we must abandon science to regain a meaningful life style? Roszak thinks not, but his vision of what our new science must be like will be unsettling to most of that fraternity, particularly those who call themselves ecologists.

> Ecology has been called the "subversive science"—and with good reason. Its sensibility—wholistic, receptive, trustful, largely non-tampering, deeply grounded in aesthetic intuition—is a radical deviation from traditional science. . . .
>
> Moreover, like all the healing arts, ecology is through and through judgmental in character. It cannot be value-neuter. Perhaps this is its most marked contrast with the other sciences. The patterns ecologists study include man in body, mind, and deed, and therefore they prescribe a standard of health. What violates the natural harmony must be condemned; what enhances it, endorsed. For the ecologist, being right means living right; the virtues of prudence, gentleness, mutual aid flow gracefully from his study. Ecology is the closest our science has yet come to an integrative wisdom. It, and not physics, deserves to become the *basic* science of the future.[31]

Although their particular emphasis differs, both White and Roszak share a conviction that it is Western man's belief system which has caused him so much grief in the technological area. Both have a faith that Western man can consciously restructure his technology if he can only bring himself to build a new set of values. While this may be a tremendously difficult undertaking, both White and Roszak assume that it can be done, and done as an act of conscious reform. Thus, however difficult the task, Western man's future still lies within his own hands.

Two Determinists: Jacques Ellul and Leslie White

Other thinkers are not as optimistic about Western man's ability to reshape his technology. The French sociologist Jacques Ellul is representative of many technological determinists who think that our freedom to control our technological environment is an illusion. In his book *The Technological Society,* Ellul says, "Primitive man, hemmed in by prohibitions, taboos, and rites, was, of course, socially determined. But it is an illusion—unfortunately very widespread—to think that because we have broken through the prohibitions, taboos, and rites that bound primitive man, we have become free. We are conditioned by something new: technological civilization." [32] Ellul uses the word *technique* to define not only mechanized, machinelike environments of Western man, but also the ways of doing things which permeate our society. Thus, technique includes computer, market research, automobile, and registration card. To Ellul, technique is all; it molds both the ideas and the actions of Western man:

> Technique integrates everything. It avoids shock and sensational events. Man is not adapted to a world of steel; technique adapts him to it. It changes the arrangement of this blind world so that man can be a part of it without colliding with its rough edges, without the anguish of being delivered up to the inhuman. Technique thus provides a model; it specifies attitudes that are valid once and for all. The anxiety aroused in man by the turbulence of the machine is soothed by the consoling hum of a unified society.[33]

Leslie White is another determinist who shares with Ellul the conviction that it is futile to believe that we really have any control over the course that Western technology will take. White's determinism is much broader than Ellul's, for in White's view it is not just technique which directs man, but the whole of culture. Some passages from White's article "Man's Control over Civilization: An Anthropocentric Illusion" will serve to illustrate his conviction that we have less say over our collective destinies than we would like to think.

> Although it is man who chips arrowheads, composes symphonies, etc., we cannot explain culture merely by saying that "man produced it." There is not a single question that we would want to ask about culture that can be answered by saying "Man did thus and so." We want to know why culture developed as it did; why it assumed a great variety of forms while preserving at the same time a certain uniformity, why the rate of cultural change has accelerated. . . . To explain all these things by saying, "Man wanted it that way" is of course absurd. A device that explains everything explains nothing. . . .
>
> You cannot explain the vast range of cultural variation by invoking man, a biological constant. In England in A.D. 1500 there was one type of culture; in Japan, another. Neither culture can be explained in terms of the physical type associated with it. . . .
>
> Nor can cultural differences be explained in terms of environment. . . . The environment of Central Europe so far as climate, flora, fauna, topo-

graphy, and mineral resources are concerned has remained constant for centuries. The culture of the region, however, has varied enormously. Here again we see the fallacy of explaining the variable by appeal to a constant.

If, then, we cannot explain cultures in terms of race or physical type . . . and if appeal to environment is equally futile, how *are* they to be accounted for and made intelligible to us?

There seems to be only one answer left and that is fairly plain—after one becomes used to it, at least. Cultures must be explained in terms of culture. . . . The culture of the present was determined by the past and the culture of the future will be but a continuation of the trend of the present. Thus, in a very real sense *culture makes itself.*

At least, if one wishes to explain culture scientifically, he must proceed *as if* culture made itself, *as if* man had nothing to do with the determination of its course or content. Man must *be* there, of course, to make the existence of the culture process possible. But the nature and behavior of the process itself is self-determined. It rests upon its own principles; it is governed by its own laws.[34]

Here, then, are two completely different philosophies. One argues that we can mold our future, can change our technology to eliminate its problems. The other argues that we have no such control. Implicit in the second view is the possibility that technological problems are probably inevitable at certain stages of cultural evolution, and the only thing we can do is to hang on and hope for the best.

As in so many broad philosophical issues of this sort, there is no way finally to resolve the question of free will versus determinism. From an evolutionary point of view, arguments can be found in support of each side. As we have noted earlier in the book, certain trends do seem to exist in evolution, and these can be interpreted as evidence that larger forces, over which we have no control, are at work. On the other hand, evolution also provides evidence for a kind of free will inherent in all life. The process of mutation is a creative one, for the new varieties which result can be unlike anything seen before. While the mutation process can be explained in rational terms, its products fall outside scientific determinism in the sense that they cannot be predicted.

Perhaps the best that any of us can do with the free-will question is to examine the arguments on each side, then make our own decisions. In any event, it seems a part of human nature to act as if we are free, even though this may be an illusion.

HOW STRONGLY IS MAN'S BEHAVIOR BOUND TO HIS BIOLOGICAL PAST?

Most of our body's physical characteristics seem to be genetically determined. They have arisen over a million or more years of organic evolution, and we have no real control over their presence or absence. Since they evolved when man was an arboreal or a hunting-gathering creature, many of these characteristics are ill adapted for Western man's technological environment.

Much of our behavior is obviously learned, rather than genetic. Our religious beliefs and politics are examples of learned characteristics, for unlike genetic characteristics, they can rapidly change. But what of behavior patterns such as aggressiveness, ambition, the urge to form a family? Are these learned or genetic characteristics? And what bearing does the answer have on a successful resolution of our technological problems? If it could be shown that most of man's behavior was genetically determined rather than learned, then we would have to proceed with great caution in our use of *any* additional technology as a means to solving our environmental and health problems. This would be so, because we would have to assume that like most of our physical characteristics, our behavioral characteristics had also evolved in a distant past, and are not adapted to a technological environment such as ours. Essentially, we would have three choices open to us if we were to be successful in creating a satisfactory environment. First, we could go back into nature—abandon our technological civilization and once again live in an environment such as that in which our body and our behavior evolved. As a second alternative, we could design a technological environment which had the basic characteristics of our old biological environment. In doing this, we would have to pay great attention to those aspects of our environment which were associated with human behavior patterns. Things such as the scale of the environment, its complexity, and its rate of change would be of vital importance, as would our social organization. A third alternative would be the drastic one of redesigning our genes to adapt them to whatever environment we wished to create.

If on the other hand it should turn out that our behavior is mostly learned and has little genetic base, then we have a much greater flexibility with regard to what we can do in manipulating our technological environment.

How much of our behavior is genetic? Just as is so for any issue, all shades of opinion can be found. Nevertheless, a tendency exists for

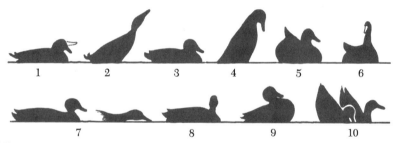

Figure 16-1. Instinctive behavior in ducks. Courtship movements of the mallard drake. Consecutive positions 1 through 10 have appearence of a learned behavior but are largely instinctive. (After Lorenz, Konrad Z., "The Evolution of Behavior," *Scientific American*, 199, December 1958, pp. 67–78.)

biologists, social scientists, and others concerned with this question to belong to one of two camps. The *ethologists* tend to see much of human behavior as instinctive, while most *social scientists* view human behavior as largely learned.

The Ethologists

Ethology is the study of animal behavior. Most ethologists are European, and most have been trained as zoologists. Typically, their work has been field-oriented; they have preferred to study animals in their natural settings rather than subject them to laboratory experimentation. Ethologists have studied all kinds of animals but have tended to concentrate on birds, fish, and insects.

Over the last fifty years, they have built an impressive case in support of their contention that a large part of the seemingly learned behavior of animals is actually genetic. During their mating season, for example, various species of birds will go through complex behavior patterns which look at if they must be learned. On closer observation, however, these turn out to be instinctive (Figure 16-1). Over the last twenty years, ethologists have begun to extend their work to include man and have become convinced that a large part of man's behavior is also instinctive rather than learned. About ten years ago, a number of ethologists began to publish their ideas in America, creating a storm of controversy which has not yet died down. They contend that such diverse behavior patterns as grooming, flirting, submissive behavior to superiors, pair bonding, and aggression all have an instinctive base. The possibility that aggression in man is instinctive has received most attention. To the ethologists aggression is a necessary instinct, one which man shares with many other species. In man, the instinct has had a particular utility, for it ensured survival when man became a hunter upon the open savannah. To ethologists, however, aggressiveness has a much broader function. As the playwright turned ethologist Robert Ardrey put it, "Aggressiveness is the principal guarantor of survival. . . . It is the innateness of the aggressive potential which guarantees that obstacles will be attacked, the young defended, new feeding grounds found when old lie waste, that orthodoxies give way to innovation when environment so demands. . . ." [35]

To many ethologists, war is aggression gone wrong. They believe that originally human aggression was ritualized. When individuals of most species aggress against each other, death rarely results. Instead, the two antagonists will face off, undergoing a series of innately determined, stylized threat postures until the weaker of the two gives in. In the human species, however, the face-to-face ritual has been lost. A bomber pilot never sees his opponent, and thus the mutual inhibitions which accompanied the old face-to-face aggression are no longer operative. As instruments of war have become more and more impersonal, killing has become greater and greater.

What arguments can the ethologists marshal in defense of their

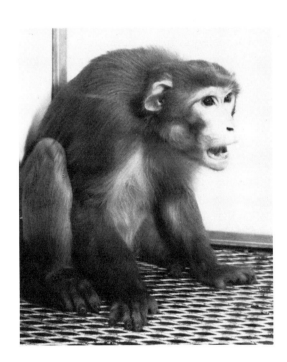

Figure 16-2. Rhesus monkey displaying aggression. (Courtesy of Harry F. Harlow, University of Wisconsin Primate Laboratory.)

views? As cited earlier, their strongest arguments come from a conviction that it is valid to extend findings made among other species to man. If instinct is strong among birds and various mammals, should it not also be found in the human species? Ethologists also base their case on the kinds of behavior that our distant ancestors most probably had. If male and female existed in pair bonds for millions of years, or if man was an aggressive hunter for a like period of time, it seems reasonable to ethologists that these behavior patterns would have become instinctive. Ethologists also use the very abnormality of life in a technological environment as evidence of their view. As Desmond Morris says in his book *The Human Zoo:*

> Under normal conditions, in their natural habitats, wild animals do not mutilate themselves, masturbate, attack their offspring, develop stomach ulcers, become fetishists, suffer from obesity, form homosexual pair-bonds, or commit murder. Among human city-dwellers, needless to say, all of these things occur. Does this, then, reveal a basic difference between the human species and other animals? At first glance it seems to do so. But this is deceptive. Other animals do behave in these ways under certain circumstances, namely when they are confined in the unnatural conditions of captivity. The zoo animal in a cage exhibits all these abnormalities that we know so well from our human companions. Clearly, then, the city is not a concrete jungle, it is a human zoo.[36]

What Morris is saying, then, is that much of what is "abnormal" in human society is so not because of some problem at the cultural level, but because of a much deeper maladjustment. Modern man has abnormal behavior because his instinctive behavioral patterns cannot adjust themselves to life in the modern technological world.

The Social Scientists

Most comparative psychologists and anthropologists take strong exception to the idea that man is such an instinctive animal. The idea that aggression is instinctive is particularly irritating to them. Here is what the American anthropologist Ashley Montagu has to say about the notion that man's aggressiveness is instinctive:

> The myth of early man's aggressiveness belongs in the same class as the myth of "the beast," that is, the belief that most if not all "wild" animals are ferocious killers. In the same class belongs the myth of "the Jungle," "the wild," "the warfare of Nature," and, of course, the myth of "innate depravity" or "original sin." These myths represent the projection of our *acquired* deplorabilities upon the screen of "Nature." What we are un-

willing to acknowledge as essentially of our own making, the consequence of our own disordering in the man-made environment, we saddle upon "Nature," upon "phylogenetically programmed" or "innate" factors. . . .

What, in fact, such writers do, in addition to perpetrating their wholly erroneous interpretation of human nature, is to divert attention from the real sources of man's aggression and destructiveness, namely, the many false and contradictory values by which, in an overcrowded, highly competitive, threatening world, he so disoperatively attempts to live. It is not man's nature, but his nurture, in such a world, that requires our attention.[37]

What evidence can be marshaled in support of the contention that little if any human behavior is instinctive?

For one thing, psychologists and anthropologists feel that ethologists depend too much on analogy. The fact that a bird or even an ape shows instinctive aggression does not mean that this behavior must also be instinctive in man. The most powerful argument in support of the social scientists' position, however, is the data from various cultures. Some primitive cultures are very warlike and aggressive; others are not. As the social scientists see it, a true instinct for aggression would imply that in *all* cultures aggression of some kind or another would exist. Furthermore, many social scientists feel that the ethologists tend to be too simplistic, to overly generalize behavioral patterns that in actuality are very complex. As Alexander Alland, Jr. says:

the existence of such intraspecific killing as homicide, infanticide, geronticide, capital punishment, war, and sacrifice demands explanation. To understand them as cultural phenomena, which indeed they are, we must not lump them under a single heading. The first four, for example, involve ingroup killing, war occurs between members of different groups, and sacrificial victims may be chosen according to custom among one's own people or among outsiders. Each type of killing has its own set of causes rooted in social life and can be understood only in the context of historical process.[38]

HOW SERIOUS IS THE TECHNOLOGICAL CRISIS IN THE WESTERN WORLD?

Has our disruption of ecosystems and our growing use of natural resources created an emergency situation? Just how much time do we have to solve these problems? Are we really less healthy than our ancestors, and if so, how serious is this problem? Once again, opinions differ.

The Environmental Crisis

In 1968 a group of industrialists, bankers, and scientists from all over the world founded the Club of Rome. The Club's purpose was to explore major issues and problems confronting modern society. The first question to which the Club addressed itself was as basic a one as can be found. What would happen to civilization if current economic and population growth rates should continue? With the aid of a grant from the Volkswagen Foundation, the Club asked an international team, headed by Dennis Meadows, an M.I.T. computer expert, to come up with answers. The team designed a computer model which simulated the interactions between such ecological variables as population growth, industrial output, natural resources, and pollution. The team fed expert opinion, factual data, and any potentially pertinent information it could find into the computer, asking this question of it: How long can the present rate of economic and population growth continue? The results were published in a book titled *The Limits to Growth*. The team stated their findings as follows:

1. If the present growth trends in world population, industrialization, pollution, food production, and resource depletion continue unchanged, the limits to growth on this planet will be reached sometime within the next one hundred years. The most probable result will be a rather sudden and uncontrollable decline in both population and industrial capacity.

2. It is possible to alter these growth trends and to establish a condition of ecological and economic stability that is sustainable far into the future. The state of global equilibrium could be designed so that the basic material needs of each person on earth are satisfied and each person has an equal opportunity to realize his individual human potential.

3. If the world's people decide to strive for this second outcome rather than the first, the sooner they begin working to attain it, the greater will be their chances of success.

These conclusions are so far-reaching and raise so many questions for further study that we are quite frankly overwhelmed by the enormity of the job that must be done.[39]

If disaster does come, just what form will it be likely to take? The computer predicted this sequence: Industrial growth would deplete natural resources, forcing industry to spend more and more of its capital on ways of using increasingly scarce resources. This would leave less and less capital free for investment in new equipment. Sometime around 2020, the world's industrial base would begin to collapse. This would involve not only a collapse of consumer goods, but of basic needs such as agricultural machinery and medical sup-

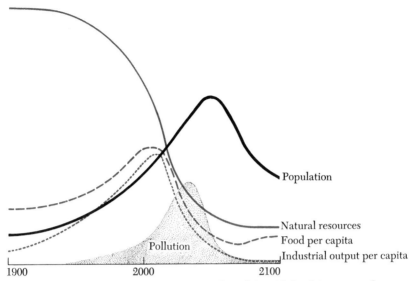

Figure 16-3. Sequence of events as predicted by Club of Rome study. Resources fail somewhere around year 2000, precipitating a world crisis.

plies. Because of this, the world's population could no longer be adequately fed or protected from disease, and a rapid population decline would take place (Figure 16-3).

The team asked the computer what could be done to avoid this global collapse. Would new, presently unknown reserves of natural resources change the prediction? What if the birth rate of the world were halved? What if food production doubled? What if pollution ended? To all such queries the computer's answer was the same. Any scenario which contains growth in population or in industry will ultimately lead to collapse of civilization as we now know it.

Other recent studies agree with the Club of Rome's conclusions. In a report titled *Blueprint for Survival,* thirty-three of the United Kingdom's most distinguished scientists foresee the same world collapse, perhaps by the end of this century. Just as does the Rome report, they see only one way out—complete cessation of both industrial and population growth.

Are the conclusions reached by the Club of Rome and by the group of United Kingdom scientists realistic, or are they overdrawn? Some scientists feel they are much too alarmist. The Rome report, for example, has been criticized as simplistic. It assumes that the world's population and its industrial growth will continue at their present exponential rate until the collapse of civilization takes place, whereas in actual fact growth rates in both areas are likely to be much more variable. Population growth rates have varied greatly in the past and certainly will not necessarily continue at an exponential rate until the next century. Actually, there are signs that population growth is already beginning to slow. Another criticism of the Rome report is that it pays too little heed to the complexities of industrial technology. For example, it may be possible to develop technologies which use entirely new kinds of raw materials, thus easing the pressure on resources which are becoming scarce.

John Maddox, who was editor of *Nature*, Britain's leading scientific journal, feels that the whole ecological crisis has been magnified beyond its real scope. In his book *The Doomsday Syndrome*, Maddox says, "The doomsday cause would be more telling if it were more securely grounded in facts, better informed by a sense of history and an awareness of economics, and less cataclysmic in temper."[40] In Maddox's view, excessive concern over the impact that Western man has had on nature may only divert attention from constructive work that needs to be done. Maddox feels that ecologists have failed to take into consideration a number of points which collectively argue that the scale of the environmental crisis has been exaggerated. Some of these points follow.

1. Man's impact on ecosystems is still relatively minor. Volcanoes and other natural agencies still have much greater power than man.

2. The problem of resource shortage has been exaggerated. Maddox notes that at the end of the nineteenth century Gifford Pinchot, a well-known conservationist of the era, "was wringing his hands over the prospect that timber in the United States would be used up in roughly thirty years; that anthracite would last for only fifty years; and that other raw materials such as iron ore and natural gas were rapidly being consumed."[41] Maddox's point is of course worth considering. Resources have had a way of stretching out, particularly as new materials are used and additional reserves of traditional resources discovered.

3. Many of the harmful effects attributed to DDT and other pollutants are either exaggerated or unproven. Maddox is particularly concerned over the way ecologists generalize in this area. He argues that just because one man-made pollutant such as DDT can be shown to harm ecosystems does not necessarily mean that all chemicals do the same thing.

4. Our population predictions have been much too simplistic.

Maddox takes strong exception to ecologists such as Paul Ehrlich, who, Maddox argues, always use the most pessimistic data available when making their predictions. As Maddox notes, many predictions assume that reproductive rates will continue unchanged at least to the end of the century yet as we noted earlier, there are signs that the reproductive rate already is beginning to decline. Maddox feels that the developing countries of the world will follow the West in moving toward a stable population, and that this transition will come much sooner than most ecologists expect. He even thinks that famine is now an "unreal scarecrow." As Maddox puts it, "There is a good chance that the problems of the 1970s and 1980s will not be famine and starvation but, ironically, the problems of how best to dispose of food surpluses in countries where famine has until recently been endemic." [42]

Although Maddox's arguments may have validity, many observers feel that it is better to err on the side of over-concern than to make the fatal error of assuming all is well when we may actually be close to disaster.

The Health Crisis

How does Western man's health compare with that of his ancestors? Unlike the issue of ecological disruption, it is not possible to identify two camps with regard to views about Western man's state of health. Instead, a number of different issues exist for which no ready answers are available. Perhaps the most difficult of these issues is this one: How do we weigh evolutionary fitness against concern for individual survival? Figure 16-4 indicates that in non-Western cultures, the less fit tend to be selected out before they have a chance to pass their genes along to the next generation. In Western culture, as represented by Japan, the technological shield allows both the fit and the less fit to reproduce. Our technology acts to save most of our citizens, regardless of any biological weaknesses they may carry or physical misfortunes they may encounter. Because of this, one could argue that we live in the most humane society the world has ever seen, at least with respect to its ability to save those human lives which earlier would have been doomed. On the other side of the picture, it may be that this is a short-sighted and temporary blessing, for as we have earlier noted it may mean that our society must support increasing numbers of individuals who carry some kind of physical handicap. Should this social burden become too great, it could disrupt and conceivably even destroy our society. One must weigh the interest of the population at large, which is to maintain a high overall fitness, against the interest of the in-

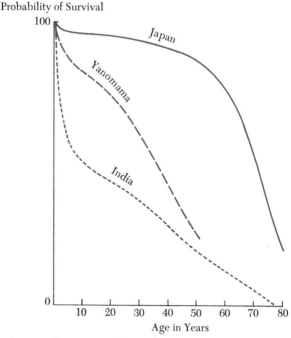

Figure 16-4. Survivorship curves for three populations. Curve of Yanomama, a primitive South American tribe, is representative of hunting-gathering man. That of India is representative of survivorship conditions which exist in advanced agricultural and early urban society. That of Japan represents modern Western technological society. (After Neel, James V., "Lessons from a 'Primitive' People," *Science,* 170 November 20, 1970, pp. 815–822.)

dividual, which is to salvage as many lives as possible through technology.

Other equally subjective issues face the person who would judge modern man's health against that of his forebears. For example, which is better, to live to forty and then die of scarlet fever as one might do in earlier times, or live to eighty, but often under conditions of chronic illness during the last twenty years of one's life?

And so we have a series of crucial questions for which no ready answers exist. In spite of this, we need to make some decisions about how to proceed in our attempts to end the disruptive effects of Western technology. Perhaps our ignorance can be of some value, for it suggests that whatever we do, we had best be cautious, acutely aware of how little we really know about the problem.

17 HOW MUCH TECHNOLOGY?

Basic to any strategy which will help us build an environment free of problems is this question: Should we invoke more technology in an attempt to solve our problems, or should we abandon the technology we have and move back toward that environment in which we evolved?

As we found in the last chapter, we are woefully ignorant in our understanding of technology. We do not know how close to disaster our technology has taken us. We do not know whether man's behavior can be adapted to a technological environment such as ours or whether it is genetically tied to the kind of environment in which our ancestors evolved. Although we act as if we have control over our technology, we are not sure whether or not this is an illusion. In the light of our ignorance over these rather fundamental questions, it would only seem prudent to proceed with great caution in creating still more technology, even though its avowed purpose may be to reduce the damage done by earlier technologies.

Evolution itself tells us to be cautious in our use of technology. As was suggested earlier in the book, all life, whether in the form of a hydra, an ecosystem, or a termite colony, is characterized by integration. Since our society is built of and for living things, we would expect it to also be integrated. Yet, in many ways, modern technology seems to be anti-life. Not only has it created problems respecting the natural environment and man's health, it has also increasingly disrupted those basic institutions which give culture its integrated character. The family has become weakened. Many of us have lost our sense of place, of belonging. Our culture is becoming increasingly fragmented into subgroups which are alienated from each other. All of these trends can be tied directly or indirectly to modern technology. Thus, it may not be too farfetched to argue that technology, which itself is an adaptive wing of man, also carries a maladaptive potential so serious as to be fatal to mankind unless we somehow curtail its tendency to disrupt our social cohesiveness.

One way to counter this trend would be to unpack most of our Western technology and deliberately (assuming, of course, that we have some control in the matter) adopt a life style similar to that of our ancestors. In this way we would be moving back toward an environment of known qualities, rather than forging ahead into the unknown and perhaps disastrous future. This is hardly a new idea. Technology, particularly machine technology, has always been looked upon with fear and distrust. Here, for example, is Samuel Butler, writing a hundred years ago in his *Erewhon,* one of the first of the anti-utopian novels:

> the machines will only serve on condition of being served, and that too upon their own terms; the moment their terms are not complied with, they jib, and either smash both themselves and all whom they can reach, or turn churlish and refuse to work at all. How many men at this hour are living in a state of bondage to the machines? How many spend their whole lives, from the cradle to the grave, in tending them by night and day? Is it not plain that the machines are gaining ground upon us, when we reflect on the increasing number of those who are bound down to them as slaves, and of those who devote their whole souls to the advancement of the mechanical kingdom? [43]

If we could somehow free ourselves of the machine and move back into a simpler life style, would our environmental and health problems solve themselves? Although there is less rebellion today against our mechanized environment than a few years ago, a large fraction of our population is attempting to do this and move our society back toward a simpler, less mechanistic way of living. This movement takes many forms. Nature communes represent one attempt to create a less technological life style; organic food diets, another. Do these movements represent the advance guard of a swelling trend, or are they instead a kind of last, nostalgic attempt to recapture our past? We think the latter is probably closer to the truth. We base our conclusion on the verdicts expressed by the American people, by other peoples of the world, and by evolution itself.

THE VERDICT OF AMERICAN SOCIETY

In a recent report, the Conservation Foundation, under contract to the National Park Service, expressed concern about trends in our national parks. Among other things, the report said:

We do not believe the Park Service is obliged to provide campsites equipped with electric outlets, running water, or toilet hook-ups. Moreover, completely modern homes on wheels are contrary to the park ethic and those who wish to use them should be asked to leave them at the park boundary and visit the park on its terms rather than theirs.[44]

While the back-to-nature faction in our culture is often outspoken, all evidence suggests that few if any Americans really wish to go back to nature, even on their camping trips.

In an amusing article titled "Daniel Boone Is Dead" David Lowenthal has this to say about the American camping public:

The general public views the outdoorsman as commendable, but seldom worth emulating. . . . Most campers today are in a hurry; they have a lot to see, and a schedule to meet. Equipment and facilities are increasingly luxurious. People with mobile trailers want electrical and water hook-ups rather than fireplaces and tables; they insist on hot and cold running water, showers, flush toilets, and laundry facilities. . . . People may like a taste of the outdoors, but they usually do not want to live in it, however briefly. Their campsites often look as unlike the outdoors as possible.

Above all, most Americans are gregarious. Solitude and silent communion with the great outdoors are the last things the average camper seeks. . . . At the Grand Canyon not one visitor in a hundred ventures below the canyon rim. Few leave well-worn paths. In Yosemite Valley, Fourth-of-July campers are estimated at more than eight thousand per square mile: "The damp night air, heavy with a pall of eye-watering smoke, is cut by the blare of transistor radios, the clatter of pots and pans, the roar of a motorcycle, and the squeals of teenagers." . . . Daniel Boone is reputed to have felt crowded when he saw the smoke from another cabin. Daniel Boone is dead.[45]

Lowenthal goes on to note that Americans do not camp so much to get away from it all as to relax in familiar surroundings. The primitive life holds little appeal for most Americans. Campers interviewed in Glacier and Quetico-Superior National Parks all expressed a love of the wilderness but also asked for more campsites and amenities.

As Lowenthal notes, most Americans like to look at, rather than live in, the wilderness. Truly wild areas are best left that way as symbols of nature, to be as little disturbed by man as possible. Even true out-

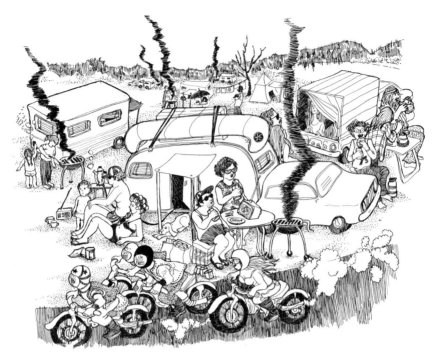

Figure 17-1. Camping American style.

doorsmen share this attitude. "We must ask even those who love the wilderness the most," says a well-known conservationist, "to touch it but seldom, and lightly." [46]

American literature can also tell us something about whether most Americans really want to return to the natural life. As the Americanist Leo Marx notes, American writers have long been fascinated by the theme of pastoralism, the withdrawal from a complex, relatively "advanced" civilization to a simpler, more natural environment. This pastoral ideal, so common in American literature, gained much of its strength from the hopes of the first settlers that a true arcadian utopia could be fashioned in the New World. However, as Marx notes, this was not to be:

> During the 19th century the image of a green garden, a rural society of peace and contentment, became a dominant emblem of national aspirations. . . . Only the most astute grasped the contradiction between the kind of society that Americans *said* they wanted and the kind they actually were creating. While the stock rhetoric affirmed a desire for a serene, contemplative life of pastoral felicity, the nation's industrial achievements

were demonstrating to all the world its tacit commitment to the most rapid possible rate of technological progress, and to an unlimited buildup of wealth and power.[47]

In the midst of this rapid evolution toward an urban technological society, a pastoral literature sprang up. Thoreau, Melville, Twain, and in our own century, Frost, Fitzgerald, Hemingway, and Faulkner all have expressed the pastoral ideal of a withdrawal to a natural environment where true peace, happiness, and order can be found. But is the pastoral ideal a true return to nature? When we look carefully at the pastoralists in American literature, two themes emerge. First, the nature which forms the pastoralist's ideal is not really nature at all. Far from being a wilderness, it is instead a rural countryside of small towns and well-tended fields. Bogs and mosquitoes are conspicuously absent. Second, in all pastoral literature, the hero's withdrawal to this pastoral utopia is inevitably followed by a return to Reality. Reality is the urban technological environment—the place, however ugly and chaotic, where the mainstream of modern civilization is still to be found.

In many other ways Americans express a certain reluctance to really return to nature. The snowmobile is a good case in point. In those parts of the country where the snowmobile is thought of as a new sort of recreational toy, feeling often runs high against its depredations

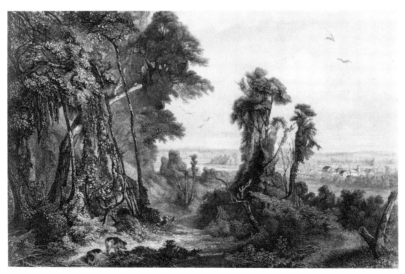

Figure 17-2. New Harmony, Indiana, a Utopian pastoral community of the 19th century. (Courtesy of the Library of Congress.)

of the natural environment. On the other hand, where snowmobiles are an economic necessity and not a luxury, attitudes are very different. In parts of northern Michigan, for example, the snowmobile has made it possible for the inhabitants to travel about, even commute to jobs which were inaccessible before. It also means winter tourists and so a new source of income in northern Michigan. He who ventures to condemn the snowmobile had best do so to himself. As one writer puts it, "It is the city dweller, divorced from a direct dependence on the land, who has taken the lead in conserving our wildlife and natural areas. Urban citizens can afford to view the eagle and coyote as beautiful creatures, not economic liabilities, and to view land they do not own or have an economic interest in as worthy of preservation in a natural state." [48]

In their camping habits, their literature, and in a thousand other ways, the great majority of Americans seem irreversibly committed to the technological life. But, one might ask, is this normal? Are Americans typical of all mankind in their preferences, or is their tendency to use nature, to remove themselves from it and then to deal with it only on their own terms a kind of cultural sickness, perhaps the result of the Christian view of nature as Lynn White, Jr. has argued?

THE VERDICT FROM THE NON-WESTERN WORLD

We suggest that all peoples, Western or not, use nature on their own terms. This is not to say that they have no respect for nature, but simply that they will take what they need from her, even if this is damaging to the natural environment, and will tend to shield themselves from her assaults as much as they possibly can. We argue that what looks like a kind of conscious conservation ethic is often a simple lack of power to take from nature. We would agree that many primitives speak of themselves as one with nature, particularly in a spiritual sense. But, as we will suggest a bit later, beliefs and needs are not always synonymous, and it is possible for a people to believe they are one with nature, yet act in a very different way.

Is there any evidence to support this view? Some does exist:

1. *Extinction of large mammals by primitive man.* As we mentioned in Chapter 7, there is considerable evidence that primitive man hunted many of the larger mammals of the world to the point of extinction.

2. *The creation of grasslands by primitive man.* Prehistoric hunters had a second major impact on the natural environment. Considerable evidence indicates that a large part of the world's grasslands may

actually be man-made. Using fire to drive animals is a time-honored way of hunting and tends to convert marginal areas into still more open space. Later, agricultural man practiced burning, both as a way of clearing land and to create fresh growth for his herds.

3. *Exhaustion of local species by primitive man.* Although he understood his local ecology in a way that Western man never has, primitive man nevertheless could still exhaust an ecosystem's natural resources. Usually, this resulted in no permanent harm to the environment, yet it could hardly be called a practice of conservationists. An example of such local depletion was given in the chapter on Bushman subsistence. Those bands which depended on the mongongo nut as a staple food would commonly exhaust local groves and be forced to travel far afield for more. In some cases of this kind, a food species seems never to have recovered from localized depletion. In certain shell middens on the California coast, the lowest levels of the midden consist of shells from one species. Higher in the midden, this species is replaced by a second species, and at still higher levels, a third species predominates. It looks very much as though the local Indians first exhausted the most desirable food species, then the next most desirable, and were finally forced to use the third variety.

4. *Disruption of the natural environment by Eastern cultures.* Although the Chinese popularly are thought of as having an almost reverent respect for nature, this did not stop them from disrupting their natural environment. As far back as the tenth century, China's forests were becoming depleted. By the last century, the north of China was largely treeless and subject to acute problems of soil erosion. Much of the forest was cut by farmers. Some was cut to deprive dangerous animals of their hiding places. Much lumber was needed for fuel and for building materials. The Buddhist practice of cremation created a heavy demand on timber resources. Finally, the civilized art of writing and the resultant need for carbon produced a drain on timber reserves. As one writer put it, "Even before T'ang times, the ancient pines of the mountains of Shan-tung had been reduced to carbon, and now the busy brushes of the vast T'ang bureaucracy were rapidly bringing baldness to the T'a-hang Mountains between Shansi and Hopei." [49]

Perhaps the most convincing evidence that all cultures serve their own interests first and nature's second comes from the results of contact between West and non-West. Whenever primitives have come into contact with the Western world, they have coveted (and the word is not too strong to use) our technology and adapted it to make more efficient use of the natural resources available to them, even though this may lead to environmental disruption. In the box entitled "Two Points of View," we describe an almost unknown tribe of Brazilian Indians. Even before direct contact with Brazilian government officials, these Indians were carving replicas of objects they wished the Brazilians to leave for them in the forest. Some objects, such as dolls,

TWO POINTS OF VIEW

The map shows a formerly isolated area of Brazil, home of an almost unknown tribe of Indians. A recently built road will open this territory to the development of the region's many resources.

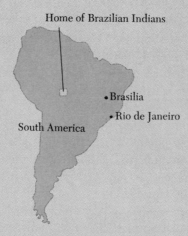

Home of Brazilian Indians

•Brasilia
•Rio de Janeiro
South America

To ease the shock that will inevitably accompany the entry of Western technology into the region, FUNAI, the Brazilian Indian agency, has established a base camp in the area. At first, the only contact between Indian and Westerner came through exchange of gifts. The agency would leave gifts hanging in the forest and in a wordless game of trust the Indians would then take these and leave their own gifts—headdresses, seeds, arrows. Some Western objects, such as scissors, knives, and needles, seemed to be more desired than others. Some were feared or resented. When toy dolls were left, they were mutilated, the bodies shot full of arrows, the heads impaled on stakes. After many months, hesitant contacts were made, and finally Indians became frequent visitors to the FUNAI base camp. These Indians will inevitably become Westernized, for in the words of one observer, ". . . there is one thing that not even the selfless, dedicated people of

were feared and rejected, but items of technology, such as scissors and knives, were sought eagerly. In our own country, the Plains Indians gladly accepted the horse, which, after all, is an object of technology. As a result, the whole Plains culture was altered. The buffalo could be hunted much more efficiently (Figure 17-3) and some students of

FUNAI can prevent. That is the erosion of a simple culture by a strong, complex one." [50]

The Tasadays (see map) are a tiny band of twenty-four stone-age

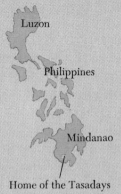

Home of the Tasadays

cave dwellers living in an almost inaccessible forest in the Philippines. Until December 1971 only one outsider, a native hunter named Dafal, had ever contacted them. Dafal taught the Tasadays to extract a nutritious starch from palm trees and introduced them to the technique of trapping animals. Before this, the Tasadays seem to have lived entirely on collected foods, such as the wild yam, tadpoles, crabs, and fish. In 1971 a government expedition (it outnumbered the Tasadays two to one!) made contact to study the life ways of this primitive group. As of this writing, the Philippine government has decided that, for the time being at least, the Tasadays should be sealed off from further change and has set aside 50,000 acres for them—a reservation large enough so the tiny band will be insulated from Western influence.

Which policy is best? To assimilate as in Brazil, or to seal off as in the Philippines? Is it morally right to take over and change a culture? What if the Tasadays don't want to remain sealed off—should they be denied the right to shatter their old culture, with all the advantages and the disruptions that will follow?

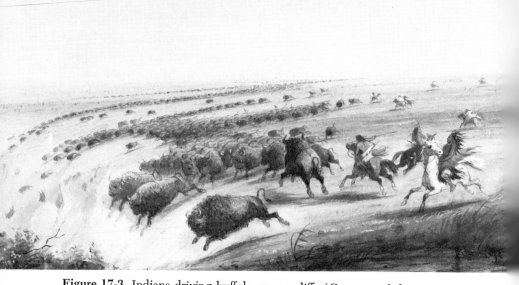

Figure 17-3. Indians driving buffalo over a cliff. (Courtesy of the Walters Art Gallery.)

Plains Indian culture feel that the buffalo would have been exterminated by the Indian had the white man never appeared on the scene. Incidentally, buffalo were hunted for much more than mere subsistence. Hides were a sign of wealth, and so more buffalo were killed than were needed for their meat. Often, only the tongue or other choice cuts were used, the rest of the animal being left to rot. Eskimos have adopted rifles and snowmobiles even though this has upset their former ecological balance with nature.

But what of the many descriptions of Indians and other primitives as conservationists? As Stewart Udall says,

> The most common trait of all primitive peoples is a reverence for the life-giving earth, and the native American shared this elemental ethic: the land was alive to his loving touch, and he, its son, was brother to all creatures. . . . During the long Indian tenure the land remained undefiled save for scars no deeper than the scratches of cornfield clearings or the farming canals of the Hohokams on the Arizona desert.[51]

How can it be that a culture will at once revere and love nature and yet despoil her? Perhaps a part of the answer to this is that man is a very complex being, capable of diverse and often contradictory behavior. As Tuan has argued, it is quite possible for a people to believe in one way, yet act in another. As he says, "A culture's publicized ethos about its environment seldom covers more than a fraction of the total range of its attitudes and practices pertaining to that environment."[52] Thus, a culture may espouse a kind of conservation ethic, but when an opportunity arises for the taking of more food or other environmental wealth, this opportunity will be exploited regardless of the idealized values of nature which are coded in the culture's belief system. All cultures seem to have this tendency to accept new technologies which give them increased power over their environment, even if this runs counter to the culture's belief system, and even if it carries the potential for ecological disaster.

If primitive peoples are so eager to accept new technology, why do they not invent it themselves? The answer to this seems to lie in the fact that technological innovation is rare in most cultures because their technology is bound to a static animism rather than to the science which drives our own innovative technology. Anthony Wiener, the futurist, calls the unique Western way of dealing with things "manipulative rationality." He says, "By 'manipulative rationality' I mean our tendency to think rationally, in terms of logical relationships of means and ends, and then to behave manipulatively, by which I mean the tendency we have to intervene in events, to act so as to change things. . . ." He then goes on to describe a hypothetical encounter between Westerner and primitive.

> Suppose you approach a man in Polynesia who is building a dugout canoe. You ask him, "What are you doing?" and he says, in effect, "I am doing the canoe building ritual." You ask, "Why are you doing it?" and he answers, "Because it's that time of the year. We've done the canoe building dance, we've sung the canoe building song, and now it's time to do the canoe building."
>
> You have manipulative rationality, you think functionally, and so you analyze the system in which he is operating and you say, "Now, aren't you really building that canoe because your people need another boat with which to go out and catch fish and bring in some more food?"[53]

Wiener goes on to point out that while the Polynesian has no difficulty in seeing that this is indeed involved, it is still not his reason for building the boat. If it were, he would be asking certain questions, such as "Should we try nets instead of boats?" or "Is there some better way to build this canoe?" He does not ask these questions, for to him boat building is not only a means to a material end but is also embedded in traditional, ritualized actions. Thus, he will continue to use the same kind of boat and the same fishing techniques for thousands of years. On the other hand, when Western technology provides him with engines to power his boats, he will accept these and increase his fishing until his fish resources threaten to become depleted.

THE VERDICT FROM EVOLUTION

As we saw in the first part of this book, all life strives to capture energy and matter, to convert these into more of its own kind. This is so for individual organisms such as a hydra; it is also true for eco-systems and for societies. Because of life's opportunism, a general evolutionary trend has taken place. Gradually, life forms have appeared which have been increasingly adept at taking matter and energy from the environment and turning these into more of their own kind. At the same time, this trend has been accompanied by a concomitant one. Those organisms most successful at energy capture are usually those which are most complex in structure and have the highest levels of integration. As judged by these criteria, man is the most advanced product of the evolutionary process. In large part, this is due to his unique position as a culture-bearing animal.

Just as do species, cultures will vary with respect to their capacity to capture energy. The anthropologist Marshall Sahlins puts it this way:

> A culture harnesses and delivers energy; it extracts energy from nature and transforms it into people, material goods, and work, into political systems and the generation of ideas, into social customs and into adherence to them. The total energy so transformed from the free to the cultural state . . . may represent a culture's general standing, a measure of its achievement.[54]

By this criterion, Western technological culture is the most advanced of any yet evolved, for its ability to capture energy far exceeds that of any other developed by man.

Assuming that energy-capture is a valid criterion of evolutionary progress, any step by Western culture back toward an earlier kind of nontechnological environment would thus be a step down the evolutionary ladder, a kind of negation of a process that embraces all life. Such a step would imply even more: It would be a renunciation of the human potential. The human species differs from all others in that only man has self-consciousness. In other species, the individuals are anonymous and serve only to perpetuate more of their own kind for generation after generation. In contrast, as a culture-bearing animal, man has the ability to plan, to dream, and to create. In the relatively short time he has been on earth, man has built a body of ideas and art, of societies and technologies that together are both his glory and his reason-to-be. In short, man is his culture. Should we strip these achievements away, only an animal would remain. While technology and the power it brings is only one part of his accomplishment, it is a vital part. As technology has increased in power and sophistication, it has acted to provide man with a material base which has freed him from animal concerns and allowed him to concentrate on purely human ones.

When used wisely, a powerful technology can create all kinds of potentials for our humanness to exploit, potentials which are denied to one who does not have access to this technology. To Arthur Clarke, Western technology's greatest contribution is the potential it gives us for exploration and adventure. In his book *Profiles of the Future* he looks at space exploration and speculates:

> The road to the stars has been discovered none too soon. Civilization cannot exist without new frontiers; it needs them both physically and spiritually. The physical need is obvious—new lands, new resources, new materials. The spiritual need is less apparent, but in the long run it is more important. We do not live by bread alone; we need adventure, variety, novelty, romance.[55]

Many of us would have uses for technology which are quite different. We might want to use its power to cure cancer, to develop a new method of restoring medieval art, of excavating underwater wrecks, or perhaps just to create satisfactory ways of existing in a steady state with nature. The point remains unchanged, however: To renounce technology is to renounce the human potential, for only technology can provide us with the material base which frees us to achieve our goals, whatever they may be.

The American citizen with his camper and the primitive with his willingness to accept Western goods both support the premise that there is to be no unpacking of our technology. The larger view of evolution also lends its support to this conclusion, for it suggests that it is inherent in life to capture more and more energy in order to build more of its own. To abandon Western technology would be, in effect, to abandon the most advanced stage in the evolutionary process.

This sweeping verdict in favor of technology is at once satisfying and ominous. As we found in Part II, as technology has evolved it has developed tendencies which seem increasingly destructive. Two of these are the destruction of the natural environment upon which man must ultimately depend, and the creation of new health problems. A third great concern is the tendency of Western technology to upset the internal integration, the sense of order and pattern of Western society itself.

The challenge is thus more demanding than most of us may realize.

Without any question, we must reform our technology in order to reintegrate it, both externally and internally. But to do this we will have to do something highly unnatural—nothing less than to remake our technology so that it no longer follows the expansionistic trend which has characterized all of evolution to date. We will examine the reasons why this must be done, and how we might do it, in the next chapter.

18

THE PROBLEM OF
TECHNOLOGICAL CHANGE

TECHNOLOGICAL FIXES

As has been emphasized throughout the book, all successful forms of life are integrated—they are in harmony with their environment and with themselves. Western technology has increasingly disrupted this integration. Part II of the book was largely concerned with showing how technology has done this in respect to our health and relationship with the natural environment. In Part II we also considered corrective technologies, or technological fixes, which have been proposed as ways of ending this disruption.

Suppose the technological fixes of Part II become a reality. What would happen? To see if we can gain some sort of answer, let's look at two of these fixes, one of which is aimed at solving a natural environment problem and the other, a health problem.

Nuclear Power

Nuclear power is likely to become an increasingly important energy source. The Atomic Energy Commission predicts that around one thousand nuclear power plants will be in operation by the year 2000. Instead of its present contribution of two per cent, nuclear power will then produce sixty per cent of our power. As we earlier indicated, nuclear power, especially fusion power, will help tremendously in solving the energy crisis.

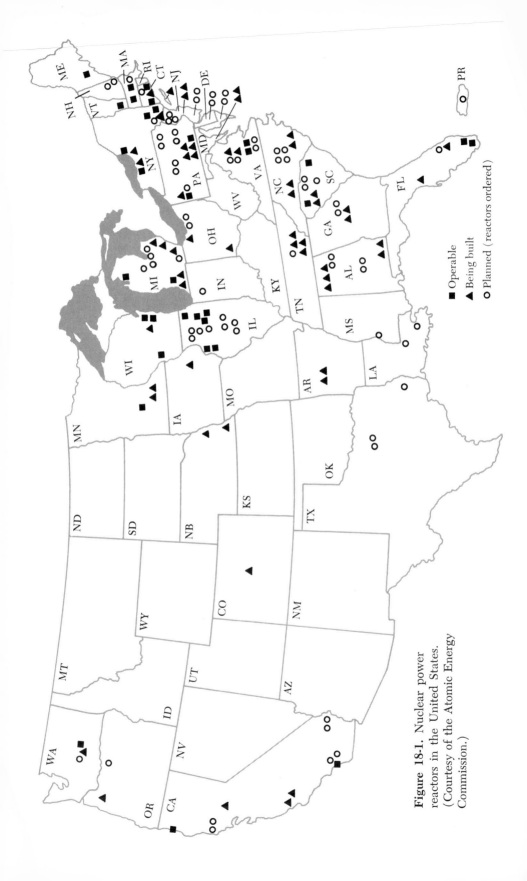

Figure 18-1. Nuclear power reactors in the United States. (Courtesy of the Atomic Energy Commission.)

■ Operable
▲ Being built
○ Planned (reactors ordered)

On the other hand, the growth of nuclear power seems likely to create a new set of problems. One of these is a health problem. Under certain conditions, it is theoretically possible for a nuclear accident to occur which would disable a nuclear power plant and release large amounts of dangerous radioactivity. How great a danger is this?

Alvin Weinberg, the former Director of the Oak Ridge National Laboratory, has this to say about the problems of nuclear plant safety:

> My main point is that nuclear plants are indeed relatively innocuous, large-scale power generators if they and their sub-systems work properly. The entire controversy that now surrounds the whole nuclear power enterprise therefore hangs on the answer to the question of whether nuclear systems can be made to work properly; or if faults develop, whether the various safety systems can be relied upon to guarantee that no harm will befall the public.
>
> The question has only one answer: there is no way to guarantee that a nuclear fire . . . will never cause harm.[56]

Weinberg goes on to argue that modern radiation technology has, however, reduced this danger to an acceptably low level. Others would disagree, and until large numbers of nuclear reactors have been built and run for many years there will probably be no answer to the question.

Nuclear power may also act to disrupt ecosystems. Nuclear generators create large amounts of waste heat, most of which is expelled in the form of hot water. Nuclear plants use about fifty per cent more cooling water than do fossil fuel plants of equal size. When a nuclear plant is through with this water, the water is also considerably hotter than the waste water produced by a conventional power plant. As nuclear energy has evolved, the waste heat problem has become increasingly important, for if it is expelled into adjacent bodies of water, this heat has the potential of completely altering existing ecosystems. Although industry and the A.E.C. are hard at work on this problem, it is far from solved.

Another problem associated with nuclear energy is that of solid waste disposal. Used fuel, which is highly radioactive, must be disposed in such a way to minimize any danger to surrounding life. To date, this has been done by holding these wastes in underground storage facilities. The latter are themselves complex technologies, consisting of tanks equipped with cooling devices which have all the potential for failure that any technology has.

Vaccines

In Part II we noted that progress is being made in an attempt to develop vaccines against the last of the great infectious diseases of the Western world. Success in the control of diseases such as influenza and the common cold would obviously be a boon to mankind, yet it would not be without its disruptive effects. Although not as important as the organic diseases, infectious diseases do account for a sizeable portion of deaths in the Western world, and eradicating these diseases would tend to further disrupt the balance of population.

The use of any vaccine to control infectious disease can lead to still another problem. When we remove ourselves from contact with the organisms of infectious disease, either through sanitary measures or through vaccination, we do not kill off all potentially dangerous organisms; we simply erect a barrier between ourselves and them. Unfortunately, this barrier makes us increasingly vulnerable to any disease organisms which are able to surmount it. This is so because our bodies come to lose the antibodies and other defenses which they carry against infection. It may even be true that our population is becoming genetically less resistant to infections, but we know little about this possibility.

Technological fixes such as those described in Part II thus have a two-faced nature. While they would solve certain problems relative to the natural environment and to man's health, they would also tend to create the potential for new problems in these areas.

We have been emphasizing the disruptive effect that modern machine technology has on the natural environment and on man's health. A point we have not emphasized is that modern machine technology has also had a disruptive effect on all of the institutions which make up Western culture. Beginning with Karl Marx, hundreds of students of our culture have concerned themselves with this problem. A large part of modern sociology is devoted to the problem of alienation, the meaninglessness and isolation felt by so many in our culture. *Anomie*, or the loss of any norms and rules one can relate to, is another problem of Western culture which has received much attention. Unfortunately, technological fixes such as those described in Part II can easily lead to still more anomie and alienation within our culture. A look at two of these fixes, population control and transplantation, will serve to illustrate how this can happen.

Population Control

One of the prime goals for Western man is to slow his rate of population growth. Suppose that through technology we succeed in achieving a steady-state population. While this would help to reduce environmental disruption, it might well increase the level of disruption in our cultural institutions. What disruptions might occur?

Amitai Etzioni, Director of the Center for Policy Research at Columbia University, has suggested some of these. In a stable population, the average age would rise and there would be fewer children or young people. This would create empty classrooms and a much larger population of retired people, both of which would produce economic problems. It might be that the birth rate among the educated and professional classes would drop more rapidly than among the poor. Etzioni believes this could intensify social conflict because there would be a larger percentage of children with few resources, who would demand their share of the West's wealth. Finally, the nation's health bill, which is already very high, would increase sharply due to the larger proportion of elderly people with chronic diseases.

Transplants

In an imaginative article, the chairman of the Department of Legal Medicine at the University of California's Medical Center has tried to imagine the disruptive effects that would follow that most bizarre of all transplants—the joining of one person's head to another person's body. The scenario goes this way: A twenty-two-year-old man, Peter Young, suffers massive brain damage in an automobile accident. On the basis of "brain death," he is declared dead shortly after admittance to Moffitt Hospital. In the same hospital lies Henry Moore, 45, victim of terminal cancer. Although his body is ridden with the disease, it has not yet reached his head. After hurried consultations, surgeons at Moffitt decapitate both patients and join Moore's head to Young's body. After the five-hour operation, the hospital reports that the patient is alive and doing well. What problems might arise? Here are a few:

1. Who is the patient?
2. How old would he be?
3. Suppose both Moore and Young had been married. Which wife is the widow? Who would receive insurance payments?
4. Would Peter Moore or Henry Young, or whoever he was, have to support both wives?
5. Genetically speaking, any offspring of Henry-Peter Young-Moore would have Young's sperm. Suppose the patient had remained with Mrs. Moore. Would "Widow Young" have a legal right to have a child by him, or at least have access to his sperm, or would this be adultery?

This sort of transplant technique is presumably still far in the future, but others with equally disturbing ramifications loom nearer. Many medical scientists think that a workable artificial heart for humans will be developed in the next ten years. A report by the National Heart and Lung Institute predicts that these will be some of the problems such a device will create:

1. Cost. Almost certainly, artificial hearts will be very expensive, perhaps costing $25,000 or more per patient. Somehow a fair financial support system will have to be created, or the device will only be accessible to the rich.

2. Who will receive the hearts? This problem, which now plagues organ transplants, will be greatly magnified. An artificial heart could save upwards of 50,000 lives a year, but it is highly unlikely that at first there will be enough to go around. Even if some kind of mass-production technology could be set up, the skills required to insert the heart would be such that medical centers staffed for the task would be overwhelmed by applicants.

3. Defining death. Once an artificial organ is inserted, particularly when it has its own power source, a new world of ethical and legal problems has been broached. Suppose it becomes possible to equip humans with both artificial hearts and brains. Suppose then that some-one's natural organs die, but his artificial heart and brain continue their functions. Is this hybrid individual dead or not? The Institute strongly

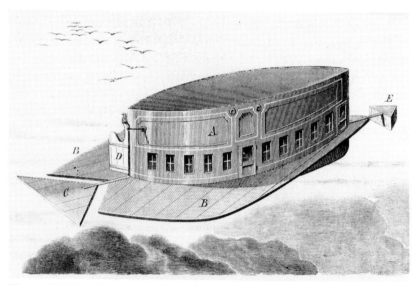

Figure 18-2. It is hard to predict what future technologies will be like, or what they will do. Proposal for an airship from *Scientific American,* July 1874. Buoyancy would be provided by a gas bag inside the ship.

recommends that we begin now to anticipate and find answers to legal and ethical problems such as these which will surely arise from artificial organ transplantation.

Perhaps the most disturbing thing about technological fixes is this: When we make forecasts about the disruptions which might ensue from nuclear power, vaccines, population control, or transplants, we are stating only the obvious possibilities. The really disruptive changes these techanological fixes might create cannot be foreseen by anyone. History provides the best evidence in support of this, for the vast changes produced by the automobile, radio, television, or other modern technologies were unanticipated. Here is one prediction which is worth pondering the next time you are caught in city traffic. It is from the July 1899 issue of *Scientific American*.

> The improvement in city conditions by the general adoption of the motor car can hardly be over estimated. . . . Streets clean, dustless, and odorless, with light rubber-tired vehicles moving swiftly and noiselessly over their smooth expanse, would eliminate a greater part of the nervousness, distraction and strain of modern metropolitan life.[57]

THE PROBLEM OF TECHNOLOGICAL CHANGE

Why is it that our technology has spawned so much disruption, and why do technological fixes seem to beget still more of the same? This disruption arises from technological change. At first, this would seem to be an absurd conclusion, particularly since we have found change to be an integral part of the evolutionary process. The disruption, however, stems not from technological change per se, but from the *rate* of change which now characterizes Western technology.

We are now in a period of technological innovation with its resulting disruption, which the biologist John Platt has called a "crisis of transformation." In an article titled "What We Must Do," Platt characterizes our problem in this way:

> There is only one crisis in the world. It is the crisis of transformation. The trouble is that it is now coming upon us as a storm of crisis problems from every direction. But if we look quantitatively at the course of our changes in this century, we can see immediately why the problems are building up so rapidly at this time, and we will see that it has now become urgent for us to mobilize all our intelligence to solve these problems if we are to keep from killing ourselves in the next few years.
>
> The essence of the matter is that the human race is on a steeply rising "S-curve" of change. We are undergoing a great historical transition to

new levels of technological power all over the world. We all know about these changes, but we do not often stop to realize how large they are in orders of magnitude, or how rapid and enormous compared to all previous changes in history. In the last century, we have increased our speeds of communication by a factor of 10^7; our speeds of travel by 10^2; our speeds of data handling by 10^6; our energy resources by 10^3; our power of weapons by 10^6; our ability to control diseases by something like 10^2; and our rate of population growth to 10^3 times what it was a few thousand years ago.

Could anyone suppose that human relations around the world would not be affected to their very roots by such changes? [58]

A good example of how the rate of change in the Western world has accelerated over the last hundred years is given by Alvin Toffler in his book *Future Shock*. Since the turn of the century, more than sixty per cent has been slashed from the time needed for a major scientific discovery to be translated into a useful product (Figure 18-3). Why is it that technological change has accelerated so? One reason is that, unlike biological change, technological change is additive. Within biological evolution, change is normally very slow. When change does

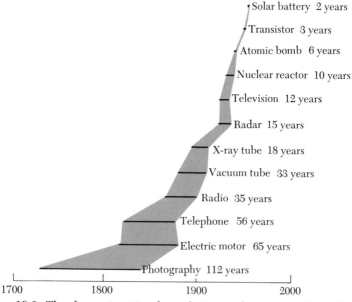

Solar battery 2 years

Transistor 3 years

Atomic bomb 6 years

Nuclear reactor 10 years

Television 12 years

Radar 15 years

X-ray tube 18 years

Vacuum tube 33 years

Radio 35 years

Telephone 56 years

Electric motor 65 years

Photography 112 years

1700   1800   1900   2000

Figure 18-3. The decreasing time-lapse between discovery and application. (After Ginsberg, Eli, *Technology and Social Change.* New York: Columbia University Press, 1964, as given in McHale, John, *The Future of the Future.* New York: George Braziller, 1969.)

appear in a life system, whether it is organism or ecosystem or insect society, it is usually selected out if it is seriously disruptive of the system's integration. In contrast, technological innovation seems to have the opposite effect; it begets still more innovation. At first, technological change was relatively slow. However, because of this property of *positive feedback* it began to gain momentum and has now attained a fantastic rate.

Two other properties of technological evolution also act to accelerate the rate at which technology changes. The first of these has to do with the way new technologies are formed. As Walter Goldschmidt and others have noted, many technological innovations are brought about by combining ideas or techniques which already exist. As the total volume of ideas and techniques in a culture increases, the ways in which these can combine will increase at a still faster rate. The second property has to do with the increasing power of technology. As this power has increased, techniques of communication have become more and more efficient, thus accelerating the rate at which technological change can spread.

Why does technological change disrupt? The following four effects seem to be involved:

1. When a new technology appears, it must be mastered. Much Western technology is highly complex. Learning to work with it, or more accurately, to get along with it, can be a stressful, disruptive process. A Bushman can master his culture's technology by the time he is twenty. Most of us understand only a tiny fraction of ours, and as new technologies appear at an increasing rate, we seem to fall further and further behind in our attempt to keep abreast of our rapidly changing technological environment.

2. When some new technology appears, it creates a wave of cultural change. These changes may involve our relationship with the natural environment, our health, our educational, economic, and political institutions, or our belief systems. Unfortunately, a new technology typically produces uneven change. Some parts of our culture may be changed drastically, other parts not at all. Many years ago, the sociologist William Ogburn labeled this tendency for different sectors of a culture to change at uneven rates *cultural lag*. This unevenness creates stress and disruption, for it weakens the integration so necessary if a culture is to function smoothly. Bushman technology was tradition-bound. Because of this, the technological changes which did appear were minor and infrequent, and could be absorbed into the culture without upsetting its integration.

3. As new technologies become more and more complex they tend to become less stable and thus more vulnerable to disruption. This is so because the very complexity of the technology means that it is prone to a greater and greater variety of breakdowns. A series of hand-dug wells, scattered across the countryside, comprises a more stable water-supply technology than a highly sophisticated, electronically controlled city water system. The latter may be much more efficient, yet because of its complexity it has many more spots of potential failure than do the hand-dug wells. Furthermore, its complexity implies a greater interdependence of units. One well can run dry and not affect others, but one failure in a computer could shut down an entire city's water-supply system. A simple lighting system such as an oil lamp is relatively stable. Failure in one household will not create failure elsewhere. In contrast, a modern power grid which supplies electric light to a city such as New York is less stable. The millions of people who were caught in New York during the great power failure of 1965 found this out in a dramatic way.

4. New technologies are increasingly associated with what Van Rensselaer Potter has called "dangerous knowledge." Two examples of dangerous knowledge would be the ability to split atoms and the knowledge of how to alter man's genes. Unfortunately, dangerous knowledge cannot be put back whence it came, although it always has the potential of creating technologies which could produce that ultimate disruption of destroying our civilization.

Damping Technological Change

In his article on the crisis of transformation, John Platt used the term *S-curve of change*. The S-curve he is talking about is depicted in Figure 18-4A. As the figure indicates, Platt feels we are now about halfway along the S and are thus approaching a point at which technological change must begin to level. But why does Platt predict an S-shaped rate of change in the first place? Why not assume that the rate of technological change will simply continue upward rather than leveling off? Evolution provides us with a convincing answer. At least to date, all living systems have followed the S-curve with respect to their rates of change. This has been so whether the system in question is a rapidly growing, expanding population of animals or a growing organism (Figure 18-4B). Thus, the feeling of many observers such as Platt is that, in one way or another, our rate of technological change must slow.

In some cases, cessation of growth and change comes about through

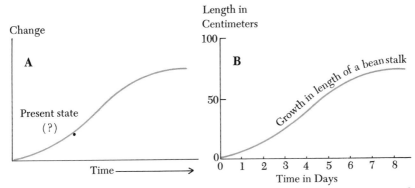

Figure 18-4. A. The general form of the S-curve of change. B. The growth curve of a beanstalk.

internal, self-regulating factors. An example of this is human maturity, when through genetic control the rapid changes associated with adolescence taper off. In other cases, however, slowing of growth or other change is brought about by pressure from external sources. In nature this often takes the form of competition from other living things. An example of leveling by external forces is the many cases of population decline brought about by famine. As suggested by the Rome Report described in Chapter 16 and by the increasing shortages of resources now facing the world, extrinsic factors beyond our control may well act to level off the West's rate of technological change. It may also be that the violence and general disruption of our time are signs that internal leveling forces over which we have no control will also work toward this end. Either sort of control will at best be unpleasant and at worst might mean the end of civilization as we know it. Certainly, a better tactic would be to try to develop alternate and more humane means of damping technological change.

How could we go about this? In part, it can be done by using still more technology. Technologies which lead to population control and to cycling of materials rather than to an ever-increasing use of natural resources would help, for they would slow the growth of our material culture. Technologies which are designed according to ecological principles also would help. Biological control of pests rather than chemical control, for example, seems to send fewer disruptive waves into natural and man-made ecosystems. Some of the more advanced medical technologies would seem to be less disruptive than more primitive ones, a possibility we will consider subsequently.

But we need to do more than this. First, we must find some way to predict what a new technology will do. As we have suggested in the last few pages, *any* technology, no matter how well-intentioned, has the potential to disrupt. Thus, we need techniques to predict coming disruption so that advance decisions can be made as to whether a given technological fix is worth it, or how it might be re-designed to minimize trouble. Secondly, it is easy to say we need to slow our rate of change. For this to occur, however, we need some means of coming to a common agreement on who does the slowing, who agrees to be the pioneer in the move toward less technological innovation. We will look at each of these problems next.

The Anticipation of Technological Disruption

Both Western technology and the Western science which lies behind much of it have always been *reductionistic*. Reductionistic thought holds that progress can only come about if a given task is disassembled so that each of its component parts can be handled separately. Our reductionistic science and technology have been highly successful. They have given us great power over nature and have freed us from many of the concerns faced by other species.

Unfortunately, reductionistic science and technology cannot predict the disruptions which ensue from new technologies. The philosopher Ervin Laszlo describes the limitations of reductionism as a method of understanding patterns of nature in the following passage from his book *The Systems View of the World.*

> Until very recently, contemporary Western science was shaped by a mode of thinking which placed rigorous detailed knowledge above all other considerations. This mode of thought was based on the implicit belief that the human mind has a limited capacity for storing and processing information. If you know some things very thoroughly, you cannot know very many different kinds of things. If you have some acquaintance with many different things, chances are you do not know them thoroughly. . . .
>
> There is one difficulty with specialization, however. This is the tendency of patterns of knowledge to create closed bubbles in their own right. Specialists in one field can communicate with one another if they share a specialty, but experience difficulty when their interests do not coincide. . . .
>
> The unfortunate consequence of such specialty barriers is that knowledge, instead of being pursued in depth and integrated in breadth, is pursued in depth in relative isolation. Instead of getting a continuous and coherent picture, we are getting fragments—remarkably detailed

but isolated patterns. We are drilling holes in the wall of mystery that we call nature and reality on many locations, and we carry out delicate analyses on each of these sites. But it is only now that we are beginning to realize the need for connecting the probes with one another and getting some coherent insight into what is there.[59]

In his book *The Closing Circle* the ecologist Barry Commoner suggests why this approach to understanding nature has led to practical problems.

Environmental degradation largely results from the introduction of new industrial and agricultural production technologies. These technologies are ecologically faulty because they are designed to solve singular, separate problems, and fail to take into account the inevitable "side-effects" that arise because, in nature, no part is isolated from the whole ecological fabric. In turn, the fragmented design of technology reflects its scientific foundation, for science is divided into disciplines that are largely governed by the notion that complex systems can be understood only if they are first broken into their separate component parts. This reductionist bias has also tended to shield basic science from a concern for real-life problems, such as environmental degradation.[60]

What kind of science and technology could overcome these limitations? An increasing number of philosophers, scientists, and technologists think that in order to successfully accomplish this vital task, we must develop a holistic or systems oriented science and technology which deals with integrated units rather than with their parts. A holistic science and technology would emphasize the integration and interrelationship between things and would thus be much more successful at anticipating the ramifications of new technologies than are our present reductionistic science and technology.

What chance is there that reductionism will be replaced by holism as our way of dealing with nature? Among our present sciences, ecology is perhaps the most holistic. In most of the biological sciences, however, thinking is still largely reductionistic and shows little sign of change. Some technologists, particularly those involved in systems work and in the new profession of futuristics think holistically, but most of technology is still reductionistic.

Agreeing to Restrain Technological Change:
The Tragedy of the Commons

In many ways, asking science and technology to reduce technological disruption is passing the buck. Until Western man can somehow reduce his desire for more and more material goods and for greater and greater variety and innovation in them, we will have technological disruption. How easily could this be done? What price, material and psychic, would we have to pay to achieve this goal?

A few years ago Garrett Hardin wrote an article which has now become a classic in ecological circles. In "The Tragedy of the Commons" Hardin pointed out a fundamental human weakness which must be overcome before any real progress can be made in stabilizing our technology. Hardin used the commons, the open pasture of an agricultural village, as an analogy to demonstrate his point. He says:

> The tragedy of the commons develops in this way. Picture a pasture open to all. It is to be expected that each herdsman will try to keep as many cattle as possible on the commons. Such an arrangement may work reasonably satisfactorily for centuries because tribal wars, poaching, and disease keep the numbers of both man and beast well below the carrying capacity of the land. Finally, however, comes the day of reckoning, that

JACOB BRONOWSKI AND THE PLACE OF SCIENCE IN A DEVELOPING ETHIC

Before we can live successfully with our technology, it may be that we must develop a new set of ethics, or rules to live by. What kind of ethics might best work in a technological society of the future? Obviously, no one yet knows. However, the thoughts of contemporary biologist-philosophers can provide us with some hints, and we present some of these in the boxes that accompany this and the next chapter.

"Every ethic looks two ways: it has a public face and a private one. That is, it must hold a man within his society, and yet it must make him feel that he follows his own free bent. No ethic is effective which does not link both these, the social duty with the sense of individuality. In this issue above all we have failed to make science part of our ethic; for we have allowed it to be pictured as a body of public knowledge and no more. As a result, we have left it to the arts to carry the private conscience that we no longer accept by edict. I have shown that neither picture is fair. Science carries its core of personal imagination too, and the knowledge of self that the arts foster reaches out to the selves of others from our own. What joins the two cultures

is, the day when the long-desired goal of social stability becomes a reality. At this point, the inherent logic of the commons remorselessly generates tragedy.

As a rational being, each herdsman seeks to maximize his gain. Explicitly or implicitly, more or less consciously, he asks, "what is the utility *to me* of adding one more animal to my herd?" This utility has one negative and one positive component.

1. The positive component is a function of the increment of one animal. Since the herdsman receives all the proceeds from the sale of the additional animal, the positive utility is nearly $+1$.

2. The negative component is a function of the additional overgrazing created by one more animal. Since, however, the effects of overgrazing are shared by all the herdsmen, the negative utility for any particular decision-making herdsman is only a fraction of -1.

Adding together the component partial utilities, the rational heardsman

and fuses them into one ethic is this double sense: the private respect for the accomplished work, the public tolerance for another man's thoughts and passions. Their conjunction is the sense of human dignity which sustains each man freely within his society, and makes him the unique and double creature: man, the social solitary. . . .

"It is the tragedy of our age that we fear the machine in man, though it is as noble as the self; and we have grown to doubt whether it will leave us a self. We will not believe that what the machine learns and teaches, a knowledge of science, can strengthen our ethic, which now languishes among our random loyalties. Yet the search for knowledge in nature generates values as rich as we get by reaching for the knowledge of self. When we pursue knowledge for action we learn (among other things) a special respect for a man's work. And when we look into another man for knowledge of our selves, we learn a more intimate respect for him as a man. Our pride in man and nature together, in the nature of man, grows by this junction into a single sense: the sense of human dignity. The ethics of science and of self are linked in this value, clarity with charity, and more than all our partial loyalties it gives a place and a hope to the universal identity of man." [61]

concludes that the only sensible course for him to pursue is to add another animal to his herd. And another, and another . . . But this is the conclusion reached by each and every rational herdsman sharing a commons. Therein is the tragedy. Each man is locked into a system that compels him to increase his herd without limit—in a world that is limited. Ruin is the destination toward which all men rush, each pursuing his own best interest in a society that believes in the freedom of the commons. Freedom in a commons brings ruin to all.[62]

The commons problem manifests itself in many ways. Every family with more than two children is taking more than its fair share of the world's resources. Strictly speaking, whenever we use a larger-than-average share of the environment, whether in the form of taking extra energy, living space, water to absorb pollutants, or whatever, we are acting as do Hardin's herdsmen.

How can we create a value system which overcomes the tragedy of the commons? One way would be to impose such a system from above, through governmental control. Let us use the population problem as an example of the kind of thing which might be done. A stable population could be attained through a variety of state-inspired controls. Some of these might be economic incentives. Payments or gifts could be made to those who accepted sterilization. "Responsibility prizes" for periods in which no children were conceived have been suggested. Heavy taxes might be levied on each child after the first two. The state could also issue "marketable licenses" to have children, with the

ALDO LEOPOLD AND THE LAND ETHIC

"All ethics so far evolved rest upon a single premise: that the individual is a member of a community of interdependent parts. His instincts prompt him to compete for his place in that community, but his ethics prompt him also to co-operate (perhaps in order that there may be a place to compete for).

"The land ethic simply enlarges the boundaries of the community to include soils, waters, plants, and animals, or collectively: the land.

"This sounds simple: do we not already sing our love for and obligation to the land of the free and the home of the brave? Yes, but just what and whom do we love? Certainly not the soil, which we are sending helter-skelter downriver. Certainly not the waters, which we assume have no function except to turn turbines, float barges, and

total in circulation just enough to keep the population at replacement level. Licenses could be bought or sold on the open market.

Other controls might be biological. Women might be sterilized by insertion of a long-lasting contraceptive, which could be removed when conception was desired. Still other controls might be social. Hardin has suggested that polyandry, the mating of several men with one woman, would effectively reduce our population. The state might encourage or even legislate a social structure of this kind.

Government control could also be invoked to manage the allocation of resources. In an Environmental Protection Agency plan recently published, automobile use would be curtailed drastically. Gas would be rationed in some areas. A limit would be put on the construction of new parking facilities. Street parking and even the use of cars in some cities would be banned. Regulations such as these would drastically reduce the number of cars on our roads and greatly help swing this particular technology toward a steady state.

The government could actively intervene in many of our technologies. Air conditioners could be restricted, the size of house lots reduced, new construction of all kinds discouraged. Various sorts of economic pressure could be put on industry to force a move toward steady-state, non-polluting, and generally less disruptive technologies. Residuals charges, or taxes on wastes, might be invoked and subsidies given to more progressive companies. As has been recently suggested, Natural Resource Units might be allocated equally to all

carry off sewage. Certainly not the plants, of which we exterminate whole communities without batting an eye. Certainly not the animals, of which we have already extirpated many of the largest and most beautiful species.

"A land ethic of course cannot prevent the alteration, management, and use of these 'resources,' but it does affirm their right to continued existence, and, at least in spots, their continued existence in a natural state.

"In short, a land ethic changes the role of *Homo sapiens* from conqueror of the land-community to plain member and citizen of it. It implies respect for his fellow-members, and also respect for the community as such." [63]

members of the population. The units would not be transferable, nor could they be bought with money. Each of us would thus have to decide how to spend his or her lifetime allocation of the world's resources.

The government could also control the use of new technology in the health area. For example, it could decide how best to allocate scarce items such as kidney machines.

Fairly obviously, the Western world is going to see an increasing amount of government control in the general area of technological use. The basic problem with such control, however, is that it tends to undermine the very benefit of powerful technology—that of providing a material base which allows men to express their individuality and follow their desires in ways never available to members of less technologically developed cultures.

A better way to damp technological change than through centralized control would be for Western man to develop a new kind of society which places less emphasis on change and the accumulation of material wealth than on ecological integration. The boxes in this and the next chapter suggest some of the characteristics that an "ethic of ecological integration" might have. Whether such an ethic could ever develop in the Western world, and if it did, whether it would be strong enough to damp technological change to an acceptable level, is one of the great questions of our time.

19 THE PROBLEM OF TECHNOLOGICAL DEHUMANIZATION

Machine technology has produced much of great value. At the same time, these values have been gained at a cost. In the last chapter we measured this cost in terms of the disruption which arises from technological change. In this chapter we consider a different kind of cost. His biological traits tell us that man is still an animal. But his cultural traits tell us that he is also much more than this. It is through his culture that man has become "human." In many ways technology is the most humane part of culture, for it is technology which releases man from the burdens of survival which form the central concern of other species and gives him the power to develop his uniquely human attributes of self-consciousness, creativity, and individuality. Yet paradoxically, it is technology, at least modern machine technology, which is responsible for much that is dehumanizing in our contemporary culture. As we noted in Chapter 17, the belief that technology is dehumanizing is hardly new. For years observers have commented on the way machine technology seems to be remaking man and his environment to emulate the values of the machine. As Siu puts it, "The Machine Age is narrowing the human response, restricting the human choice, and depersonalizing the human virtues. Like a hermit crab shaping its body to the conformity of the dead shell it has picked up, social patterns today are being molded along the confines of soulless machines." [64]

Theobald notes that we increasingly use the machine metaphor in our everyday lives. He says:

Listen to the repetition of the machine metaphor in these colloquial expressions:

Let's run this proposal through the mill.
The news media act as a conveyor belt for government propaganda.
The economy has built up a head of steam; let some steam out of it.
Toss that idea into the hopper.
That meeting was like going through a grinder.
Step on the gas and get moving.
Run him out on a rail.
This thing runs like clockwork.
He engineered the victory.
He's a big wheel.
That man is just a cog in the wheel.
Be careful or he'll steamroller you.
You want to throw a monkey wrench into the works? [65]

Perhaps former Mayor Lindsay of New York best stated our uneasy feeling that machines are molding us in their image when he said, "I just think the question comes down to this: What is a city for? Is it for people, or is it for automobiles and the gasoline engine? Unless people win out in this struggle, the city won't be livable, and no place will be livable." [66]

This dominance of machine over human values is thus the second kind of technological problem we wish to deal with.

THE DEHUMANIZING EFFECT OF TECHNOLOGY

The Scale of a Machine Environment

The ethnologist Desmond Morris opens his book *The Human Zoo* in this way:

Imagine a piece of land twenty miles long and twenty miles wide. Picture it wild, inhabited by animals small and large. Now visualize a compact group of sixty human beings camping in the middle of this territory. Try to see yourself sitting there, as a member of this tiny tribe, with the landscape, your landscape, spreading out around you farther than you can see. No one apart from your tribe uses this vast space. It is your exclusive home-range, your tribal hunting ground. Every so often the men in your group set off in pursuit of prey. The women gather fruits and berries. The children play noisily around the camp site, imitating the hunting techniques of their fathers. If the tribe is successful and swells in size, a splinter group will set off to colonize a new territory. Little by little the species will spread.

Imagine a piece of land twenty miles long and twenty miles wide. Picture it civilized, inhabited by machines and buildings. Now visualize a compact group of six million human beings camping in the middle of this territory. See yourself sitting there, with the complexity of the huge city spreading out all around you, farther than you can see.

Now compare these two pictures. In the second scene there are a hundred thousand individuals for every one in the first scene. The space has remained the same. Speaking in evolutionary terms, this dramatic change has been almost instantaneous; it has taken a mere few thousand years to convert scene one into scene two.[67]

The dramatic change in scale described by Morris has come about almost entirely as a result of machine technology. The machine's power and efficiency has directly led to the huge aggregates which we call cities. Is the scale of our modern culture, as represented by the city, inhuman? Ethologists such as Morris are convinced that many of Western man's problems are directly related to the fact that he has simply not had time to adapt to the massive scale of this new environment. Many students of man would disagree with the notion that our culture's troubles might be due to genetic maladaptation, but almost all agree that the massive scale of a machine culture has had a disruptive and dehumanizing effect on modern man. As the scale of our environment increases, that of the individual decreases. Modern man lost in a huge, impersonal society is a common theme in Western literature today. When our cultural institutions increase in scale, they seem to become less and less sensitive to the dignity and individuality of those people whom they are supposedly serving. Paul Goodman, the late social philosopher, described this as it applied to penal institutions:

as technology increases, as there is a proliferation of goods and as civilization becomes more complex, there is a change of the scale on which things happen. Then, if we continue to use the concepts that apply to a smaller scale, we begin to think in deceptive abstractions. There are certain functions of life that we think we are carrying on, and that *were* carried on on a smaller scale, but which now on a larger scale are only seemingly being carried on. Sometimes, indeed, because of the error in our thinking, we get an effect opposite from that which was intended.

Consider penology, a poignant example. When some fellows sat in stocks in the town square and people passed by and jeered at them or clucked their tongues, it is possible, though the psychology is dubious, that the effect might have been reform or penitence. (In my opinion,

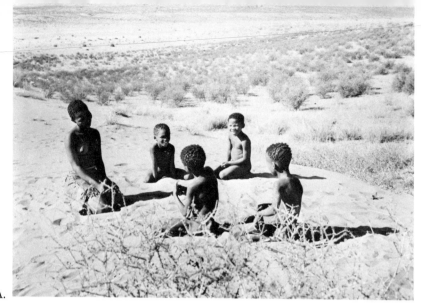

A.

Figure 19-1. A. Bushmen in the veld. Natural environments such as the veld have surrounded man for 99% of his time on earth; the man-made environment, for less than 1%. (Courtesy of the South African Information Service.) B. A totally human engineered environment, the Pan Am Building in midtown Manhattan. (Courtesy of the New York Convention and Visitors Bureau.)

B.

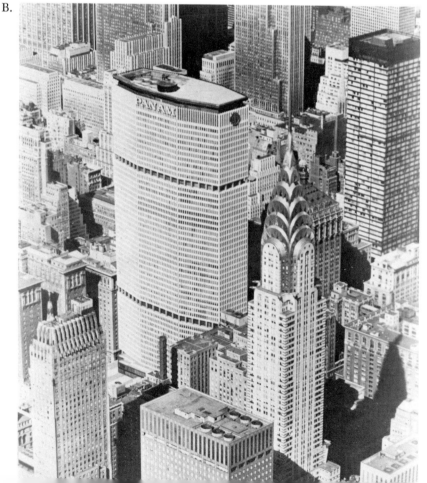

public confession on the square was more likely to lead to penitence and social integration.) But the Tombs in New York, a jail for many thousands locked up in cages, obviously has no relation whatever to penitence, reform, or social integration. In fact it is a school for crime, as is shown by the rate of repeaters who come back on more serious charges. This kind of penology on this scale has the opposite effect from that intended: it produces crime. Yet we have come by small steps from the fellow in stocks on the town square up to the Tombs or San Quentin. It seems to be "penology" all along the line, but there has been a point at which it has ceased to be penology and has become torture and foolishness, a waste of money and a cause of crime. And even the social drive for vindictiveness, which is probably the chief motive for punishment, is not satisfied; instead, there is blotting out of sight and *heightening* of social anxiety.[68]

Goodman goes on to cite similar effects in the areas of education, the media, and medicine. In each case, the huge scale of these institutions has made them less and less responsive to the needs of individuals in our society.

In her book *The Death and Life of Great American Cities* Jane Jacobs has argued persuasively that the violence so common in our urban renewal housing projects is due primarily to their scale. Most of these developments consist of huge high-rise buildings containing hundreds of identical apartments. Great care is taken to segregate these from areas of commercial, industrial, business, educational, or recreational activity. Living in one of these developments is all too often a dehumanizing experience. The scale of the buildings creates anonymity and kills any sense of belonging. Residents often do not even know their neighbors and certainly not those who occupy other floors. Because all functions other than simply providing a place to live have been eliminated from the buildings, they are often half deserted. The sum effect is to isolate people and create areas for crime. Stairwells, even halls, become places of danger, to say nothing of the lonely, parklike expanses of green which often surround these developments.

Jacobs argues that many older city neighborhoods, which superficially appear run-down and dangerous, are actually much safer and more human places to live. This is so because in these neighborhoods residences, shops, schools, and other activities are all mixed together. One result of this is that the scale of living is much reduced—people know each other in such a neighborhood. In addition, the diversity of activities means that many people are coming and going, so someone is always on hand to keep an eye on things and prevent crime or other violence. Interestingly, Jacobs' ideal city neighborhood can be thought of as resembling a natural ecosystem in its diversity, small scale, and stability, while in its large scale, lack of diversity, and instability, an urban housing development resembles a modified cultural ecosystem such as a wheat field.

When we talk about change in scale, we usually think in terms of an increase in some dimension, but the change can also be one of decrease. Culminating a process which began with the advent of agriculture, machine technology has created an urban society. In the crowded cities typical of Western technology, people tend to have less and less privacy. What Edward Hall has termed our space bubbles—our personal chunks of the environment—have been steadily reduced in scale, for we have become increasingly pressed by other people, either physically as on a crowded street, or verbally, through the immense volume of information we receive via the media. Is this kind of crowding or density in our life style dangerous? Some biologists think that it is.

Around fifteen years ago John Calhoun used rats to demonstrate the idea that extreme crowding could indeed lead to pathology in living things. In his experiments Calhoun used pens arranged as shown in Figure 19-2. Each pen was a complete dwelling unit, with abundant food, water, and places to nest. As shown in the figure, ramps were arranged so that all but pens I and IV were connected. Calhoun placed one or two pregnant females in each pen and awaited developments. Young were born and mated to produce more young. As the density of

PIERRE TEILHARD DE CHARDIN AND A PURPOSEFUL WORLD

"The world is a-building. This is the basic truth which must first be understood so thoroughly that it becomes an habitual and as it were natural springboard for our thinking. At first sight, beings and their destinies might seem to us to be scattered haphazard or at least in an arbitrary fashion over the face of the earth; we could very easily suppose that each of us might *equally well* have been born earlier or later, at this place or that, happier or more ill-starred, as though the universe from the beginning to the end of its history formed in space-time a sort of vast flower-bed in which the flowers could be changed about at the whim of the gardner. But this idea is surely untenable. The more one reflects, with the help of all that science, philosophy and religion can teach us, each in its own field, the more one comes to realize that the world should be likened not to a bundle of elements

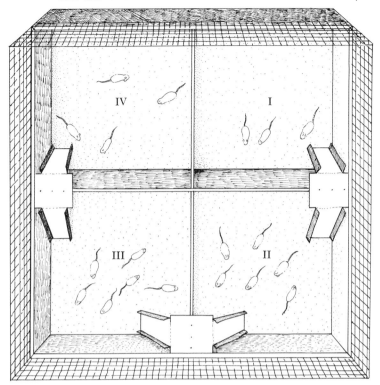

Figure 19-2. Experimental arrangement of pens used by Calhoun. Details in text.

artificially held together but rather to some organic system animated by a broad movement of development which is proper to itself. As the centuries go by it seems that a comprehensive plan is at work in the universe, an issue is at stake, which can best be compared to the processes of gestation and birth; the birth of that spiritual reality which is formed by souls and by such material reality as their existence involves. Laboriously, through and thanks to the activity of mankind, the new earth is being formed and purified and is taking on clarity and definition.

"Now, we are not like the cut flowers that make up a bouquet; we are like the leaves and buds of a great tree on which everything appears at its proper time and place as required and determined by the good of the whole." [69]

the rat population increased, a sorting-out process took place. Pens I and IV were each occupied by a dominant male, who maintained a harem of about ten rats and kept all other males from entering. This was relatively easy to do since each pen had only one access ramp. Fourteen less dominant males plus a number of females thus were forced to crowd into pens II and III. As new rats were born, these pens became more and more crowded, and abnormal behavior began to develop. Some males became sexually hyperactive, attempting to chase and mount any other animal, whether male or female. Other males became withdrawn and almost completely inactive. The females in pens II and III built abnormal nests and failed to raise their young properly.

A number of other studies which have been performed after Calhoun's classic work have added to the suspicion that overcrowding produces behavioral pathology, probably as a result of an overtaxed stress system. The crucial question for us is of course whether a continuing increase in human density could also lead to pathological behavior. Doubters point to the fact that man can exist under many levels of density and still carry out apparently normal behavior. Believers argue that much of the city violence which we ascribe to other causes may actually be a result of dense living conditions. Although one study suggests that crime, juvenile delinquency, and other pathologies among

PERRY LONDON AND AN ETHIC OF AWARENESS

"In what respect should men be free to engage other people cooperatively, antagonistically, or not at all? . . .

"The contemporary version of this ancient problem differs from early ones in some important details which sharpen its focus but do not change its fundamental character. First, as society becomes progressively more technical and complex, it may also be more delicate and vulnerable to bottlenecks and breakdowns, so that anyone who removes himself from it or rebels against it may endanger the welfare or survival of everyone else more than at any time in the past. Second, more powerful means exist today than ever before for coercing social responsibility. Third, and most important here, behavior-control technology makes it possible not only to rationalize coercion in terms of the common good but also to engineer individual consent. . . .

"The only deterrent or reply to behavior control is to increase (man's) technical mastery of his own behavior. Man's shield and buckler and

city people may be related to density per se rather than to education, economic level, or other causal factors, the density thesis has yet to be proven.

The Standardization of a Machine Environment

Machine technology has created a much greater variety of things than ever was present in any primitive culture. After all, any small-town hardware store contains literally thousands of different items, and our total material culture must be composed of literally hundreds of thousands of different kinds of objects. This variety is, of course, one of the great dividends of an affluent machine technology, for it has given man the power of choice. Yet, paradoxically, the same machines which create variety have acted to diminish uniqueness. To illustrate this, consider an object such as a knife. Our technology must produce several thousand different kinds of knives, whereas only one or two kinds can be found in a primitive culture such as the Bushman's. On the other hand, my pocket knife is exactly like a million others of its kind. If I lose it and later find a knife of the same kind, I may have considerable difficulty telling whether it is indeed my old knife. In contrast, although a Bushman's knife has a general resemblance to all other Bushman knives, it also has a uniqueness that is lacking in my

finally, his most potent weapon, is his individual power of awareness.

"With this the case, we then must ask what ethical prescriptions follow from this ideology. If ideology does not mean just ideas, but ideas to be acted on, what actions do the ethics of awareness demand? There are at least four. Of technology, it demands that individual development be maximized and people provided with the instruments of self-control; men must know their tools. Of politics, it demands that men be free and the machinery of government forever vulnerable to individual action against it; men must have their rights. Of free men, it demands that they be conscious of the need to share the world with other men and exercise restraint on their own willfulness; men must know some limits. Of society, it demands that it renounce coercion as its chief instrument of control and substitute persuasive means which individuals may finally take or leave, even at some peril to us all; men must take some risks." [70]

knife. Since a Bushman makes his own knife, it directly reflects his unique needs and artistic abilities. I may have a wider variety of knives to choose from, but no matter which knife I choose it will be an impersonal thing, formed by an anonymous machine in some anonymous factory. Machine made objects may relieve me of a certain drudgery, but at the same time they have a dehumanizing effect, for they deprive me of the sense of pride, satisfaction, and even power that comes to him who has the ability to create his own environment.

We may laugh at the thought of returning to a handicraft technology, but hobbies, gardening, even the do-it-yourself movement, bespeak a widespread urge to recapture a personal participation in the creation of material things, which the machine has taken away.

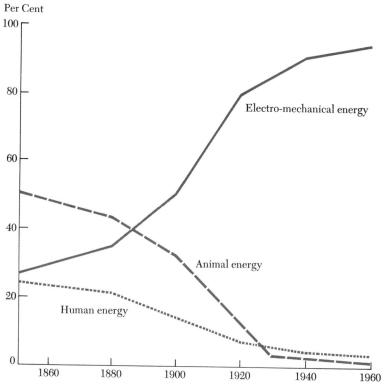

Figure 19-3. Rise in electro-mechanical energy during the last hundred years. The shift to electro-mechanical energy implies a shift to an impersonal, anonymous kind of energy, as compared to that provided by animals or man himself.

There are many different ways in which the machine takes away uniqueness, to replace it with standardization, a value much closer to its own metallic heart. Many foods now are quantified and made uniform through the power of machine technology. In his book *Man and Food* Magnus Pyke tells how our machine technology has even quantified and standardized the "crunch" of food. A technician chews various crunchy foods such as toast or celery. While doing so, he wears a hearing-aid-like instrument, which picks up and records the frequency and amplitude of his chewing sounds. From this information, decisions can be made as to how crunchy a given kind of food should be. Once this decision is made, production techniques can be developed to ensure that all lots produced have a uniform crunch.

Standardization of this sort is of great value to machines, for it helps them to carry out their tasks efficiently. While such standardization does help machines to produce a greater quantity of food for man, it has a dehumanizing effect, for it threatens to eliminate the variety of textures, tastes, sights, and smells which have always been a part of man's food. As van Dresser puts it, "All the old lusty smells and sensations attendant upon the grinding of corn, roasting of coffee, the fermenting of yeast in bread or beer, the pressing of apples or grapes, have been banished in favor of a hushed operating room asepsis." [71]

The evolution away from nature and into the standardized world of the machine permeates all of our environment. Again, in van Dresser's words, "In this careful cosmetic world there are no gnarled people, no mature or older men and women whose faces, bodies and hands have been formed and indented through direct contact with the brines, caustics and tannins of elder nature. . . . In this environment, no balance of the physical, the intellectual and the esthetic may be expected to evolve." [72]

Some writers feel that the machine and its strivings toward standardization are now acting to reduce the *total* variety of things produced by our machine technology. According to Kenneth E. F. Watt:

Textural and cultural diversity has declined in our cities, whether you compare different parts of the same city or different cities in different countries. Driving from an airport to the downtown section of a city, the signs tend to be in the same language (English) and to advertise the same products, whether one is in Rome, Beirut, or Singapore. Stores and banks seem to be stamped from a common mold.

Remarkably, the same process has occurred in the human population. An extraordinarily high proportion of the world's population is now very young. The variety once found when many human age classes coexisted in approximately equal numbers has gone.

There are too many examples of the decline of diversity for this situation to have come about by chance. There is indeed an underlying explanation: we live in an age, and a culture, that puts tremendous emphasis on efficiency and productivity as desiderata for mankind. Since variety is inimical to these goals, variety has suffered and will continue to suffer. Unless powerful and compelling arguments can be offered to stop this loss of diversity, we will soon be living in a homogeneous—and boring—world.[73]

It would be more than a dehumanized, boring world. In evolutionary terms, it would be a dangerous one, for all of evolutionary history argues that those life forms which are most diverse have had the greatest chance for survival. This has been so for two reasons. First, as we found in comparing natural and cultural ecosystems, diverse systems are more stable than simplified ones. Second, diverse systems are better equipped to cope with new and unexpected evolutionary challenges than are simplified ones, for they are more likely to carry internal variants which are adapted to the new challenge.

Many parts of the Western world thus far have managed to resist the standardized environment produced by a machine technology. In her article "Reading the Roof-Lines of Europe" May Theilgaard Watts has caught the sense of variety and adaptation to local conditions which much of Europe's rural housing still shows. In the Po Valley of Italy, "Roofs take on added responsibilities. The tiled roofs of the two-story farm-houses stretch out into an 'L' shape. One wing of the house accommodates cattle downstairs and the family upstairs, and is provided with an outside stairway. The other wing is open, except for its roof and one side, which is built up with open-work brick lattice. The open wings are empty in June, but are stuffed to capacity with baled hay in late summer, before the rainy season." Alpine houses form a sharp contrast. "Here the spreading roofs hold thick chunks of slate used for shingles, and boulders used to anchor the slates against the wind; and thick feather-beds of snow for additional warmth. The eaves are wide. They spread like the wings of a brooding hen. Travelers are glad to find refuge from rain under their spread; and to eat lunch under their shelter; and later to fall asleep listening to their slow drip in the foggy night." In Denmark and in England, "many cottages wear their roofs like stockingcaps, pulled low around their ears. The use of thatching indicates an abundance of moisture, which reduces the danger of fire in those roofs which would otherwise be so vulnerable. These roofs accompany beech forests, and velvet lawns and tall spikes of delphinium that last for days and days in that cool humidity." And how does she characterize American roof lines? "They offer no comment on wind, or rain, or local quarries, or forests. They speak only of style and solvency. A roof has become only another piece of merchandise, as unrelated to environment as its owner's creased trousers. . . ." Unfortunately, as she points out, "Such progress will not be denied to Europe. It will reach quickly from Normandy to Provence and the Black Forest and Denmark; and then climb more slowly to the hill towns, and to the Alps, and Norway; and then creep across the moors of Scotland." [74]

Machine Man

In a culture dominated by machines, it is only natural that man himself comes to be thought of as a machine. While many would have strong reservations, most biologists would probably agree with Dean Wooldridge when he says man is no more than a complex machine, or even with Buckminster Fuller's imaginative and disturbing description of man as

> a self-balancing, 28-jointed adapter-base biped, an electro-chemical reduction plant, integral with the segregated stowages of special energy extracts in storage batteries, for subsequent actuation of thousands of hydraulic and pneumatic pumps, with motors attached; 62,000 miles of capillaries, millions of warning-signal, railroad, and conveyor systems; crushers and cranes . . . and a universally distributed telephone system needing no service for 70 years if well managed; the whole, extraordinarily complex mechanism guided with exquisite precision from a turret in which are located telescopic and microscopic self registering and recording range finders, a spectroscope, et cetera.[75]

Most experimental work in human biology rests on the assumption that the human body can be explained in machine terms; indeed, the whole structure of experimental science as applied to man must make this assumption. The investigations of man-as-machine now have evolved to the point where once mysterious and forbidden areas of humanness are being penetrated and exposed as explicable in ordinary mechanistic terms. Increasingly, it looks as if the brain and even the elusive thing we call consciousness can be so explained. Recent experiments with rats have suggested that memory is a mechanistic process. Rats were taught to avoid the dark, then sacrificed, and an

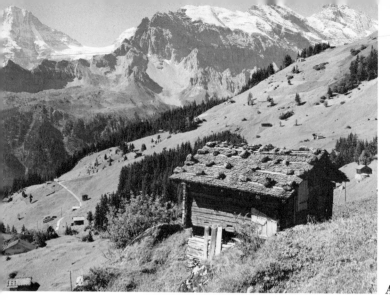

A.

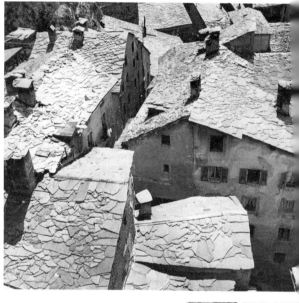

B.

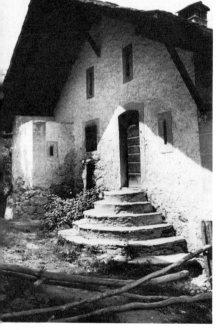

C.

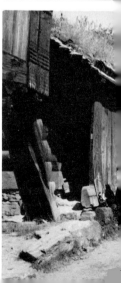

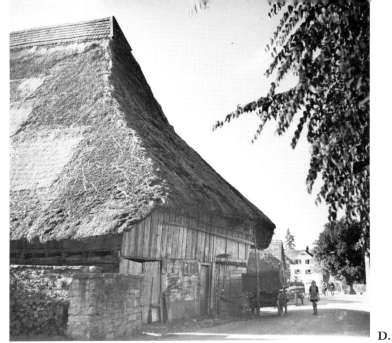

D.

E.

Figure 19-4. Houses in Switzerland: (a) Above the village of Mürren in the Bernese Oberland; (b) shingle roofs of houses of Sion in the Valais Valley; (c) a wide-eaved peasant home in the Valais; (d) a straw-roofed farmhouse in Lenzburg. (Courtesy of the Swiss National Tourist Office.) Houses in Norway: (e) A stave church; (f) grass roofs of reconstructed ancient buildings in a park of the Norwegian Folk Museum in Oslo. (Courtesy of the the Norwegian National Travel Office.)

F.

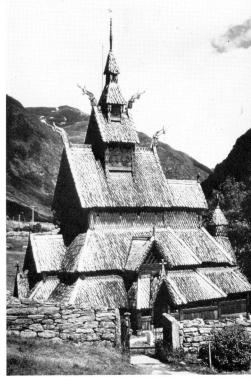

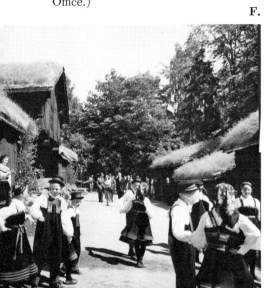

extract of their brains injected into other untrained rats. The latter then acted as though they also had been trained. According to those who conducted the experiment, the "memory molecule" which they managed to identify in the extract was a protein that apparently had been synthesized in the brains of the trained rats and then passed along to the untrained ones.

A good deal of experimental work has shown that certain human emotions can be controlled through tiny electrodes placed within the brain. In a series of spectacular experiments, José Delgado of Yale and other researchers have been able to manipulate the emotions of mentally disturbed people. A number of investigations have suggested that such generalized behavior patterns as a baby's love for its mother can be profitably studied, using a mechanistic approach. Harry Harlow and his associates at the University of Wisconsin Primate Laboratory have found that young monkeys need a certain set of characteristics in the object they perceive as "mother." When these are withheld, the infant will develop into an abnormal adult. In this work, surrogate mothers of cloth and wire were used to test the attributes a mother must provide for its offspring to develop normally.

As is true for all things our machine technology has done, the concept

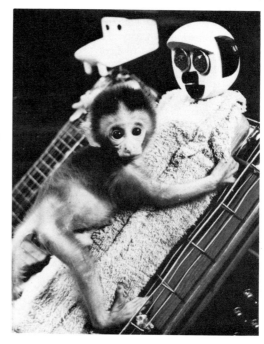

Figure 19-5. Harry F. Harlow and his associates at the University of Wisconsin have shown that bodily contact is a primary motive in attracting a baby to its mother. In the photo, the rhesus monkey is clinging contentedly to a surrogate mother of soft cloth. (Courtesy of Harry F. Harlow, University of Wisconsin Primate Laboratory.)

of man-as-machine has been both beneficial and at the same time harmful. On the positive side, great insight has been gained into the workings of the human body, and the way has been opened for management of diseases, both physical and mental. On the other hand, if men are viewed as machines, it is only a short step to *treat* them as such. The work of José Delgado, for example, has opened the possibility that we may be able to build humans of our own design. As Delgado says, "We're very close to having the power to construct our own mental functions. . . . The question is what sort of humans would we like, ideally, to construct?" [76]

The attitude that man is some sort of machine, open to manipulation or redesign, has increasingly permeated our biological circles. This has led to many promising medical technologies, such as those described in Part II of this book. Unfortunately, it has also led biological research to use man as a "guinea pig"—a subject for experimental research. Recently, much controversy has arisen over the use of convicts as experimental material in the testing of new drugs. It is not uncommon for medical researchers to use terminal patients for experimental purposes. In one case of hospital experimentation, live cancer cells were injected into twenty-two patients as part of a study of immunity to cancer. The patients were not told details of the experiment. When questioned as to whether he would have used himself as a subject, one of the investigators was reported to have replied, "if it would have served a useful purpose. . . . I do not regard myself as indispensable—if I were not doing this work someone else would be . . . and I did not regard the experiment as dangerous. But let's face it, there are relatively few skilled cancer researchers, and it seemed stupid to take even the little risk." [77]

The view of man-as-machine creates all kinds of problems when death grows near. Since modern medical technology now has the ability to prolong the act of dying, the physician, the family, and even the patient, if he is responsive, face a set of bewildering problems. As Leon Kass, who is executive secretary of the Committee on the Life Sciences and Social Policy, National Research Council, National Academy of Sciences, has said:

> Certain desired and perfected medical technologies have already had some dehumanizing consequences. Improved methods of resuscitation have made possible heroic efforts to "save" the severely ill and injured. Yet these efforts are sometimes only partly successful; they may succeed in salvaging individuals with severe brain damage, capable of only a less-than-human, vegetating existence. Such patients, increasingly found in the

intensive care units of university hospitals, have been denied a death with dignity. Families are forced to suffer seeing their loved ones so reduced, and are made to bear the burdens of a protracted death watch.[78]

If death is a mechanical thing, a mere stoppage of the human machinery, what particular failure marks its appearance? A large literature is accumulating over this problem, but no ready solutions seem to be in sight.

In another, very different way, our mechanistic approach to man's ills has had a dehumanizing effect. The very complexity of modern medical technology tends to diminish the patient and make him feel lost within a maze of mysterious and sometimes frightening machinery. Again in Kass' words:

> Even the ordinary methods of treating disease and prolonging life have impoverished the context in which men die. Fewer and fewer people die in the familiar surroundings of home or in the company of family and friends. At that time of life when there is perhaps the greatest need for human warmth and comfort, the dying patient is kept company by cardiac pacemakers and defibrillators, respirators, aspirators, oxygenators, catheters, and his intravenous drip. [79]

CREATING A HUMANE TECHNOLOGY

In his epic work *Technics and Civilization* Lewis Mumford saw Western technology as evolving through three stages. The first of these

RENÉ DUBOS AND THE OPEN FUTURE

"The cynics, or those who consider themselves realists, can in fairness point out that searching for a new faith that would unite society is like chasing a will-o'-the-wisp. Many kinds of philosophical, social, and religious faiths have appeared in the course of history, only to disappear like shooting stars consuming themselves in the sky. . . .

"Why, then, speak of national purpose, social purpose, or any kind of purpose? . . .

"As I write these lines two contrasting pictures come to my mind, one of a juvenile delinquent, the other of a painting by Daumier.

"The fundamental characteristic of the true juvenile delinquent is that he acts only for the sake of the present, for the satisfaction of an urge, of an appetite, or of a whim. He has not learned that man differs from animals by consciously relating the present to the future; indeed,

was the Eotechnic. This was the technology of Medieval Europe, with its wind and water power. The next stage, the Paleotechnic, began in the eighteenth century and reached its culmination in the last decades of the nineteenth. Of all technologies, the Paleotechnic seemed most inhuman to Mumford. Iron and coal became predominant resources. Cities became grim, blackened with soot, and filled with crowded slums. Life became increasingly quantified, and its tempo sped up to keep pace with machines. People became objects, mere resources used to man the mines and factories which sprang up everywhere. Hours were long, work often mechanical and carried out under the worst of conditions. When he wrote *Technics and Civilization,* in the 1930's, Mumford anticipated that the Paleotechnic era would be replaced by a new level of technological evolution, the Neotechnic. In the Neotechnic, electricity would be the dominant form of energy. Light metals and plastics would replace the iron and steel of the Paleotechnic. Through automation, man would escape the dehumanizing work of the Paleotechnic. In short, the Neotechnic would become an era in which man once again recaptured his humanness, stolen from him by Paleotechnic excesses. Much of our present-day technology fits Mumford's description of the Neotechnic, yet technology seems to be as much and probably more of a problem than ever. In his later writing, Mumford has tended to be less of an optimist respecting the ease with which we can bend technology to our interests. Yet the ideal remains— that with hard work, a change in values, and a good deal of luck, a more humane technology can be created.

he has no vision whatever of the future. In contrast, the masterpiece by Daumier, *The Uprising,* seems to be a symbol of human willingness to struggle for the future. This painting, in the Phillips Gallery in Washington, shows a vigorous and handsome young man on a barricade with outstretched arms and clenched fists. His visionary gaze is lost in the distance toward a future that he will never know, because he will not live long enough; bullets will probably soon strike him down. Certainly it is a vague future that the revolutionary on the barricade sees in his imagination; at most it means Liberty, perhaps Equality and Fraternity. Daumier's hero is the symbol of *Man,* the animal with an open future which he creates through faith in the human condition. He's the eternal nomad of the questioning spirit, haunted by the future and blind to danger, the eternal standard-bearer of a worthwhile cause." [80]

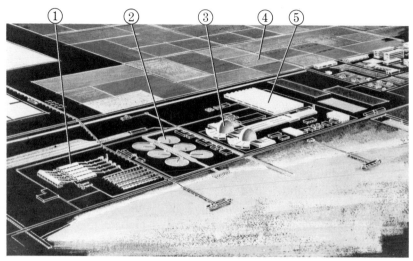

Figure 19-6. Agro-industrial complex: (1) electric furnace and phosphorous plant; (2) seawater treatment plant; (3) reactors; (4) scientifically managed farms, and (5) aluminum fabrication.

Creating a Humane Environmental Technology

Figure 19-6 shows an agro-industrial complex of the sort envisioned by many agricultural technologists. In such a complex, nuclear reactors would generate millions of kilowatts of energy. This power would be used to desalt water for irrigation, make fertilizer, run factories, and produce crops. The whole complex would feed about six million people. A hundred thousand farmers, factory workers, and their families would live in the complex.

This vision of the future symbolizes a great triumph of Western man, for it typifies the imaginative, powerful, and efficient technology created through his long struggle to subdue the environment about him. At the same time, it also symbolizes a failure, for individuals have somehow become lost in this massive, complex, and standardized technology.

Figure 19-7 shows an "ecological house" designed by Grahame Caine, an English architectural student. Organic wastes from the household are used to fertilize vegetables and fruits grown in the garden and to produce methane gas for cooking. The house is warmed by solar heat, and additional energy would come from wind-generated power in winter. Grahame Caine's house can also stand as a symbol, but in this case of a new and rehumanized environmental

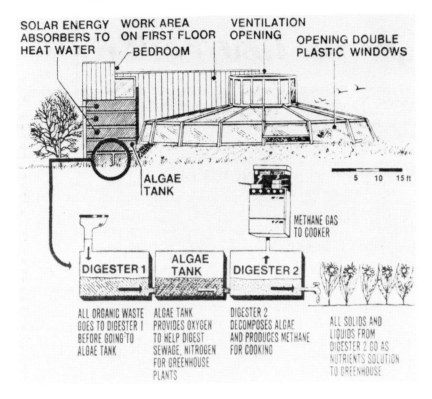

SOLAR ENERGY ABSORBERS TO HEAT WATER

WORK AREA ON FIRST FLOOR — BEDROOM

VENTILATION OPENING

OPENING DOUBLE PLASTIC WINDOWS

5   10   15 ft

ALGAE TANK

METHANE GAS TO COOKER

DIGESTER 1

ALGAE TANK

DIGESTER 2

ALL ORGANIC WASTE GOES TO DIGESTER 1 BEFORE GOING TO ALGAE TANK

ALGAE TANK PROVIDES OXYGEN TO HELP DIGEST SEWAGE, NITROGEN FOR GREENHOUSE PLANTS

DIGESTER 2 DECOMPOSES ALGAE AND PRODUCES METHANE FOR COOKING

ALL SOLIDS AND LIQUIDS FROM DIGESTER 2 GO AS NUTRIENTS SOLUTION TO GREENHOUSE

Figure 19-7. An ecological house designed by Grahame Caine, an English architectural student. (*The London Observer.* Reprinted with permission of *Los Angeles Times/Washington Post* News Service.)

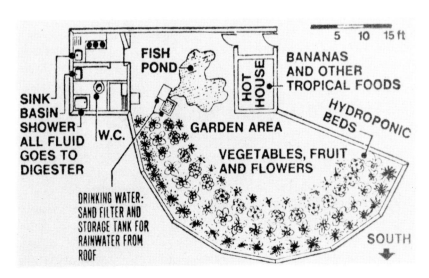

5   10   15 ft

FISH POND

BANANAS AND OTHER TROPICAL FOODS

HOT HOUSE

SINK BASIN SHOWER ALL FLUID GOES TO DIGESTER

W.C.

GARDEN AREA

HYDROPONIC BEDS

VEGETABLES, FRUIT AND FLOWERS

DRINKING WATER: SAND FILTER AND STORAGE TANK FOR RAINWATER FROM ROOF

SOUTH

technology. Here, the technology has been scaled down, it has re-gained a human dimension. As envisioned by Caine, each ecological house would be designed to reflect the particular needs and interests of its owner; each would be unique. Caine's house was designed specifically to reduce reliance on large-scale alienating technologies such as the agro-industrial complex and to replace them with a human-scale technology run by and reflecting the needs and interests of individuals.

Creating a Humane Health Technology

Doctor Lewis Thomas, Dean of the Yale University School of Medi-cine, characterizes our present health technology as "highly sophisticated and at the same time profoundly primitive." Dr. Thomas uses con-temporary management of coronary disease as an example of such a "half-way technology." He says:

> An extremely complex and costly technology for the management of heart disease has evolved, involving specialized ambulances and hospital units, all kinds of electronic gadgetry, and whole platoons of new professional personnel to deal with the end results of coronary thrombosis. Almost everything offered today for the treatment of heart disease is at this level of technology, with the transplanted and artifical hearts as the ultimate examples.[81]

What would a humane health technology be like? As with humane environmental technologies, it would no longer resemble the coronary disease technology Dr. Thomas describes, which dwarf its human users in power, scale and complexity. What might stand as a symbol of this new kind of health technology? Perhaps the biofeedback tech-niques now being explored, for they minimize the machine and maximize the role of one's own body as the prime mover in health management.

How Can We Build Humane Technologies?

1. *Through more science.* In spite of the dangers involved, a humane health technology can only be brought about through the use of still more science. Not until we have developed a more profound under-standing of man and his body can we learn how to effectively control disease without the use of a massive, alienating technology. In Dr. Thomas' words, and again using coronary disease as an example, "When enough has been learned to know what really goes wrong in heart disease, we ought to be in a position to figure out ways to prevent or

reverse the process; and when this happens, the current elaborate technology will be set to one side." [82]

In a similar fashion, we will need more science to achieve a humane environmental technology. One of the great dilemmas of the technologies such as envisioned by Grahame Caine is that they are less efficient in the production of wealth per person than are the large-scale standardized technologies of the agro-industrial kind. If we are not to forsake the wealth and its attendant potential for variety, comfort, and even challenge which our present machine technology has provided us, we must learn how to make our environmental technology at once less dehumanizing, yet at the same time maintain its efficiency.

Is this too utopian a dream? Some feel it is, and argue that return to a more humane environmental technology will inevitably be accompanied by a lower material standard of living. Others, such as Buckminster Fuller, one of the most influential thinkers of our time, do not agree. Fuller says:

> My own picture of humanity today finds us just about to step out from amongst the pieces of our just one-second-ago broken eggshell. Our innocent, trial-and error-sustaining nutriment is exhausted. We are faced with an entirely new relationship to the universe. We are going to have to spread our wings of intellect and fly or perish. . . .
>
> We begin by eschewing the role of specialists who deal only in parts. Becoming deliberately expansive instead of contractive, we ask, "*How* do we think in terms of *wholes*?" [83]

Fuller goes on to say that through the use of systems theory, of a sane and realistic use of materials, and of man's unique ability to progress in understanding, we can fashion an environment that is both humane and productive of wealth.

2. *Through a system of values which bring man and machine into proper balance.* To Lewis Mumford, both our current preoccupation with technology and our concept of man as primarily an energy-capturing species reflects a dangerous misconception. As Mumford sees it:

> Art and technics both represent formative aspects of the human organism. Art stands for the inner and subjective side of man; all its symbolic structures are so many efforts to invent a vocabulary and a language by which man became able to externalize and project his inner states, and most particularly, give a concrete and public form to his emotions, his feelings, his intuitions of the meanings and values of life. Technics, on the contrary, develop mainly out of the necessity to meet and master the external con-

ditions of life, to control the forces of nature and to expand the power and mechanical efficiency of man's own natural organs, on their practical and operational side. Though technics and art have at various periods been in a state of effective unity—so the fifth century Greeks, for example, used the word technics to apply both to fine art and utilitarian practice, to sculpture and stonecutting—today these two sides of culture have split wide apart.[84]

To Mumford, modern man's greatest problem is that of restoring a balance between art and the machine. He says:

> I believe that the relations between art and technics give us a significant clue to every other type of activity. . . . The great problem of our time is to restore modern man's balance and wholeness: to give him the capacity to command the machines he has created instead of becoming their helpless accomplice and passive victim; to bring back, into the very heart of our culture, that respect for the essential attributes of personality, its creativity and autonomy, which Western man lost at the moment he displaced his own life in order to concentrate on the improvement of the machine.[85]

How does Mumford propose to restore this balance? In part, the problem is a political one. In his most recent book, *The Pentagon of Power,* Mumford argues that our culture puts an overemphasis on technology because it is used to further the interests of a totalitarian power system. Yet the problem is also a personal one, resident in all of us. And what is the solution to this problem? Something we should have been aware of from the beginning:

> We have gratuitously assumed that the mere existence of a mechanism for . . . mass production carries with it an obligation to use it to the fullest capacity. *But there simply is no such necessity. Once you discover this, you are a free man.*[86]

20 _____THE DISTANT FUTURE

If the near future is difficult to foresee, the distant future is much more so. What does the far evolutionary future have in store for man? Unless we have been completely misled by the evolutionary process, we can anticipate further change in man's condition. But what kind of change? Here are two views, which lie at opposite ends of a continuum of possibilities.

TEILHARD AND THE OMEGA POINT

A Jesuit priest, the late paleontologist-philsopher Pierre Teilhard de Chardin developed a unique view of man's place in the evolutionary process. Essentially, Teilhard saw evolution as leading toward ever greater degrees of complexity, interaction, and consciousness. He saw the evolutionary process as passing through a series of levels; matter, life, thought, and society, the latter being the level occupied by modern man. Teilhard thought newer levels evolved from earlier ones by a process which consisted of an initial expansion and radiation, followed by consolidation and then evolution to the next level. After life appeared, it first underwent a period of slowly increasing volume and diversity. At some point in this process, the intensity of life became such that a consolidation, or *involution*, began. Living things began to interact with each other at increasing intensities. Finally, a critical point was reached which led to the creation of the next level, thought. A similar process of consolidation and interaction then produced the present level which Teilhard called the social.

Much of Teilhard's work is couched in a terminology which is seen by many biologists as far too mystical and spiritual to be called scientific. For example, Teilhard talks about life as "groping," with an

THE LIMITS OF PERCEPTION

In his book *The Invisible Pyramid* Loren Eiseley asks us to imagine that we are a single white blood cell trying to understand the nature of its universe, namely the body that it inhabits.

"The cell would encounter rivers ramifying into miles of distance seemingly leading nowhere. It would pass through gigantic structures whose meaning it could never grasp—the brain, for example. It could never know there was an outside, a vast being on a scale it could not conceive of and of which it formed an infinitesimal part. It would know only the pouring tumult of the creation it inhabited, but of the nature of that great beast, or even indeed that it was a beast, it could have no conception whatever. It might examine the liquid in which it floated and decide, as in the case of the fall of Lucretius's atoms, that the pouring of obscure torrents had created its world.

"It might discover that creatures other than itself swam in the torrent. But that its universe was alive, had been born and was destined to perish, its own ephemeral existence would never allow it to perceive. It would never know the sun; it would explore only through dim tactile sensations and react to chemical stimuli that were borne to it along the mysterious conduits of the arteries and veins. Its universe would be centered upon a great arborescent tree of spouting blood. This, at best, generations of white cells, by enormous labor and continuity, might succeed in charting.

"They could never, by any conceivable stretch of the imagination, be aware that their so-called universe was in actuality the prowling body of a cat or the more time-enduring body of a philosopher, himself engaged upon the same quest in a more gigantic world and perhaps deceived proportionately by greater vistas." [87]

How much of reality can we perceive? Is it possible that our images of reality are as far from the truth as those of Eiseley's thinking cell?

Here are some arguments in support of this possibility.

"inner principle" and a drive which explains its "irreversible advance" toward higher levels.

What did Teilhard see as the ultimate fate of man? Since he saw evolution as a continuing process, this could only mean the emergence of yet another level to follow the "social level" that we now occupy. To Teilhard, the increasing importance of communication in modern

1. Our sense receptors are limited. For example, the electromagnetic energy spectrum (see the figure) runs all the way from very long TV waves to very short gammas. Yet we can sense only a thin slice of this spectrum, that which we call "visual." In a similar way, our senses of sound, smell, and touch are limited, and ESP suggests we may be completely ignorant of some very important aspects of reality.

2. What we think we see "out there" is strongly conditioned by our past experience. The sense of perspective is largely learned, and blind people who have regained sight must learn to make sense of their surroundings, for at first they see nothing but a spinning mass of light and color.

3. Evidence from physics suggests that every time we observe some objects about us the very act of observation distorts those objects.

All this suggests that our ability to perceive the future must forever be limited, not only by our incomplete understanding of those forces which shape the evolutionary process, but also by the finite nature of our perceptions.

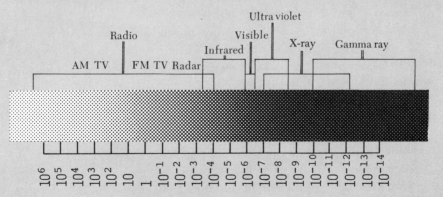

Wavelength in Meters

The electromagnetic spectrum, showing the wavelengths which correspond to various electromagnetic radiations.

society is a sign that involution toward the next evolutionary level is now under way. Teilhard thought that the next level would be marked by a kind of collective consciousness, a merging of the minds of all men into one "interthinking unit." At the same time, individual personalities would retain their integrity, a rather difficult combination to visualize. Teilhard saw the ultimate goal of the evolutionary process as a union of all things into an "Omega point," which many readers of Teilhard interpret as a godlike principle. Interestingly, Teilhard saw the Omega point as the answer to the entropy problem which we posed at the beginning of this book:

> In Omega, we have . . . the principle we needed to explain the persistent march of things toward greater consciousness . . . (a gravitation) against the tide of probability toward a divine focus of mind which draws it onward. Thus something in the cosmos escapes from entropy, and does so more and more.[88]

CLARKE AND THE ASCENDANCY OF THE MACHINE

A number of futurists, of which Arthur Clarke is an example, have built quite a different future for man. In their view, one fact stands out above all others: A slow but inevitable evolution toward machine dominance is taking place. Already machines can do many, if not most, of the things men can do. They can move about, think after a fashion, and store and retrieve information at a rate far superior to our limited abilities.

To Clarke, it seems inevitable that the skills of machines will continue to increase and that we will become even more dependent on them than we now are. Most of our dependency will be at an impersonal level, such as is true when we rely on machines to process business records or the like. However, it seems likely that our personal behavior may also become increasingly dependent on machines. One example of how this might happen is provided by OLIVER, the On-Line Interactive Vicarious Expediter and Responder, a computer planned to relieve us of many personal decisions. OLIVER would store a huge variety of personal information for its owner. Items such as food preferences, likes and dislikes of one's friends, important dates, even personality traits, could be stored in OLIVER. In addition, OLIVER would be tied into public data pools containing information such as weather predictions or the current behavior of the stock market. Properly programmed, OLIVER could make simple decisions for its owner, and might even sit in for its owner at committee meetings or similar functions, drawing on its coded information to make the same responses its owner would make to any given situation. Without too much stretch of the imagination, one could visualize a group of OLIVERs resolving simple problems without human intervention.

In still another way machines may come to play an increasingly intimate role in our lives. *Cyborgs,* or man-machine hybrids, are becoming more and more common. A person on a kidney machine is a kind of cyborg, as would be the thousands who would use artificial hearts should they be perfected. Clarke predicts that man's increasing intimacy with his machines will have an inevitable outcome: Man will become obsolete and thus be discarded. He says:

> If this eventually happens—and I have good reasons for thinking that it must—we have nothing to regret, and certainly nothing to fear. . . . No individual exists forever; why should we expect our species to be immortal? Man, said Nietzsche, is a rope stretched between the animal and the superhuman—a rope across the abyss. That will be a noble purpose to have served.[89]

Although many of us would take issue with Clarke's vision of man's eventual obsolescence, few of us would dispute this description he gives of man as an insignificant waystop along the vast reaches of evolution:

Our Galaxy is now in the brief springtime of its life—a springtime made glorious by such brilliant blue-white stars as Vega and Sirius, and, on a more humble scale, our own Sun. Not until all these have flamed through their incandescent youth, in a few fleeting billions of years, will the *real* history of the universe begin.

It will be a history illuminated only by the reds and infrareds of dully glowing stars that would be almost invisible to our eyes; yet the somber hues of that all-but-eternal universe may be full of color and beauty to whatever strange beings have adapted to it. They will know that before them lie, not the millions of years in which we measure the eras of geology, nor the billions of years which span the past lives of the stars, but years to be counted literally in trillions.

They will have time enough, in those endless aeons, to attempt all things, and to gather all knowledge. They will not be like gods, because no gods imagined by our minds have ever possessed the powers they will command. But for all that, they may envy us, basking in the bright after-glow of Creation; for we knew the universe when it was young.[90]

FOOTNOTES

1. Eugene S. Schwartz, *Overskill* (Chicago: Quadrangle, 1971), pp. 4, 7.
2. Philip Handler, "The Federal Government and the Scientific Community," *Science,* **171:** 147–148 (January 15, 1971).
3. Cited in George Gaylord Simpson, *Biology and Man* (New York: Harcourt, 1966), p. 21.
4. Dean E. Wooldridge, *Mechanical Man* (New York: McGraw-Hill, 1968), p. 167.
5. Mary J. Marples, "Life on the Human Skin," *Scientific American,* **220:** 108 (January 1969).
6. Cited in Leslie A. White, *The Science of Culture* (New York: Farrar, 1949), p. 87.
7. Ashley Montagu, *The Human Revolution* (New York: Bantam, 1967), p. 76.
8. Elizabeth Thomas, *The Harmless People* (Baltimore: Penguin, 1969), pp. 145–146.
9. Ibid., pp. 111–112.
10. Ibid., p. 19.
11. Ibid., p. 88.
12. James V. Neel, "Lessons from a 'Primitive' People," *Science,* **170:** 819 (November 1970).
13. R.G.H. Siu, *The Tao of Science* (Cambridge: M.I.T. Press, 1966), p. 48.
14. Mary Ann Spencer Pulaski, *Understanding Piaget* (New York: Harper, 1971), pp. 167–168.
15. I. I. Rabi, *Science: The Center of Culture* (New York: World, 1970), p. 130.

16. Roger L. Welsch, *Sod Walls* (Broken Bow, Nebraska: Purcells, 1968), p. 146.
17. John B. Jackson, "Ghosts at the Door," *The Subversive Science*, (Boston: Houghton, 1969), p. 160.
18. Edgar Anderson, *Plants, Man and Life* (Berkeley: U. of Cal., 1967), pp. 136–137, 141.
19. Cited in Donald W. Coon and Robert R. Fleet, "The Ant War," *Environment*, **12:** 30 (December 1970).
20. Cited in Marston Bates, "Man as an Agent in the Spread of Organisms," *Man's Role in Changing the Face of the Earth* (Chicago: U. of Chicago, 1965), pp. 799–800.
21. H. S. Glasscheib, *The March of Medicine* (London: MacDonald, 1963), p. 119.
22. Ibid., p. 125.
23. Peter van Dresser, "The Modern Retreat from Function," *The Subversive Science* (Boston: Houghton, 1969), p. 367.
24. Jean Mayer, *Overweight* (Englewood Cliffs, N.J.: Prentice-Hall, 1968), p. 79.
25. Cited in Stanley Milgram, "The Experience of Living in Cities," *Science*, **167:** 1461 (March 13, 1970).
26. Victor Papanek, *Design for the Real World* (New York: Pantheon, 1971), p. 62.
27. H. J. Muller, "Human Evolution by Voluntary Choice of Germ Plasm," *Evolution of Man* (New York: Oxford, 1970), p. 543.
28. Lynn White, Jr., "The Historical Roots of our Ecologic Crisis," *Science*, **155:** 1205 (March 10, 1967).
29. Ibid., p. 1205.
30. Ibid., p. 1207.
31. Theodore Roszak, *Where the Wasteland Ends* (Garden City, N.Y.: Doubleday, 1972), pp. 400–401, 413.
32. Jacques Ellul, *The Technological Society* (New York: Vintage, 1967), p. xxix.
33. Ibid., p. 6.
34. Leslie White, op. cit., pp. 338, 339, 340.
35. Robert Ardrey, *The Social Contract* (New York: Delta, 1971), pp. 258–259.
36. Desmond Morris, *The Human Zoo* (New York: McGraw-Hill, 1969), p. 8.
37. M.F. Ashley Montagu, "The New Litany of 'Innate Depravity' or Original Sin Revisited," *Man and Aggression* (New York: Oxford, 1968), p. 16.
38. Alexander Alland, Jr., *The Human Imperative* (New York: Columbia U. P., 1972), p. 31.
39. Donella H. Meadows et al., *The Limits to Growth* (New York: Universe, 1972), pp. 23–24.
40. John Maddox, *The Doomsday Syndrome* (New York: McGraw-Hill, 1972), p. 4.
41. Ibid., p. 6.
42. Ibid., p. 5.

43. Cited in John G. Burke, ed., *The New Technology and Human Values* (Belmont, Cal.: Wadsworth, 1966), pp. 9–10.
44. Michael J. Conlon, "Trailer, Car Park Ban Urged," *The State Journal* (Lansing, Mich.: September 17, 1972), p. A-4.
45. David Lowenthal, "Daniel Boone Is Dead," *Natural History Magazine*, 47: 11 (August–September 1968).
46. Ibid., p. 9.
47. Leo Marx, "Pastoral Ideals and City Troubles," *The Fitness of Man's Environment, Smithsonian Annual II* (Washington, D.C.: Smithsonian Institution Press, 1968), p. 126.
48. Daniel A. Guthrie, "Primitive Man's Relationship to Nature," *BioScience*, 21: 722 (July 1, 1971).
49. Cited in Yi-Fu Tuan, "Our Treatment of the Environment in Ideal and Actuality," *American Scientist*, 58: 248 (May–June 1970).
50. W. Jesco Von Puttkamer, "Brazil Protects Her Cinta Larga Indians," *National Geographic*, 140: 424 (September 1971).
51. Stewart Udall, *The Quiet Crisis* (New York: Avon, 1967), p. 16.
52. Tuan, op. cit., p. 244.
53. Anthony J. Wiener, "Faust's Progress: Methodology for Shaping the Future," *Shaping the Future* (Amsterdam: North-Holland, 1972), pp. 49, 50.
54. Marshall D. Sahlins and Elman R. Service, eds., *Evolution and Culture* (Ann Arbor: U. of Mich., 1970), p. 35.
55. Arthur Clarke, *Profiles of the Future* (New York: Bantam, 1971), p. 83.
56. Alvin M. Weinberg, "Social Institutions and Nuclear Policy," *Science*, 177: 29 (July 7, 1972).
57. Cited in Robert Theobald, *Habit and Habitat* (Englewood Cliffs, N.J.: Prentice-Hall, 1972), p. 44.
58. John Platt, "What We Must Do," *Science*, 166: 1115 (November 28, 1969).
59. Ervin Laszlo, *The Systems View of the World* (New York: Braziller, 1972), pp. 3–4.
60. Barry Commoner, *The Closing Circle* (New York: Knopf, 1971), p. 193.
61. J. Bronowski, *The Identity of Man* (Garden City, N.Y.: Natural History Press, 1966), pp. 106–107.
62. Garrett Hardin, "The Tragedy of the Commons," *Science*, 162: 1244 (December 13, 1968).
63. Aldo Leopold, *A Sand County Almanac* (New York: Oxford, 1968), pp. 203–204.
64. Siu, op. cit., pp. 128–129.
65. Theobald, op. cit., p. 43.
66. "A Street Without Cars," *The New Yorker*, 49: 23 (July 2, 1973).
67. Morris, op. cit., pp. 11–12.
68. Paul Goodman, "Two Points of Philosophy and an Example," *The Fitness of Man's Environment, Smithsonian Annual II* (Washington, D.C.: Smithsonian Institution Press, 1968), pp. 27–28.
69. Cited in Robert Francoeur, *Evolving World, Converging Man* (New York: Holt, 1970), pp. 198–199.

70. Perry London, "The Ethics of Behavior Control," *Readings on Ethical and Social Issues in Biomedicine* (Englewood Cliffs, N.J.: Prentice-Hall, 1973), pp. 165, 166, 172, 173.

71. van Dresser, op. cit., p. 364.

72. Ibid., pp. 366, 367.

73. Kenneth E.F. Watt, "Man's Efficient Rush Toward Deadly Dullness," *Natural History*, **81**: 75 (February 1972).

74. May Theilgaard Watts, "Reading the Roof Lines of Europe," *The Subversive Science* (Boston: Houghton, 1969), pp. 169, 173, 174, 176.

75. Cited in Lewis Mumford, *The Pentagon of Power* (New York: Harcourt, 1970), p. 56.

76. Maggie Scarf, "Brain Researcher José Delgado Asks—'What Kind of Humans Would We Like to Construct?'," *New York Times Magazine*, November 15, 1970, p. 46.

77. Henry K. Beecher, "Medical Research and the Individual," *Life or Death, Ethics and Options* (Seattle: U. of Wash., 1968), p. 142.

78. Leon R. Kass, "The New Biology: What Price Relieving Man's Estate?" *Science*, **174**: 784 (November 19, 1971).

79. Ibid., p. 784.

80. René Dubos, *The Torch of Life* (New York: Simon & Schuster, 1970), pp. 128–129, 130.

81. Lewis Thomas, "Guessing and Knowing: Reflections on the Science and Technology of Medicine," *Saturday Review*, **55**: 55 (December 23, 1972).

82. Ibid., p. 55.

83. R. Buckminster Fuller, *Operating Manual for Spaceship Earth* (New York: Simon & Schuster, 1972), pp. 52–53.

84. Lewis Mumford, *Art and Technics* (New York: Columbia U. P., 1968), pp. 31–32.

85. Ibid., p. 11.

86. Ibid., p. 100.

87. Loren Eiseley, *The Invisible Pyramid* (New York: Scribners, 1970), pp. 33–34.

88. Pierre Teilhard de Chardin, *The Phenomenon of Man* (New York: Harper, 1965), p. 271.

89. Clarke, op. cit., pp. 226–227.

90. Ibid., pp. 231–232.

BIBLIOGRAPHY

These books have been chosen for one or more of the following reasons: readability, novel approach to the subject, classic statement of the topic, or availability.

The reader is also directed to the books cited in the Footnotes.

Man, Life, and Evolution

BERTALANFFY, LUDWIG VON. *Problems of Life*. New York: Harper and Row, Publishers, Inc., 1960.

CRICK, FRANCIS. *Of Molecules and Men*. Seattle: University of Washington Press, 1970.

LANGLEY, L.L. *Homeostasis*. New York: Van Nostrand Reinhold Company, 1965.

MUNSON, R. (ed.). *Man and Nature*. New York: Dell Publishing Co., Inc., 1971.

SAVAGE, JAY M. *Evolution*. New York: Holt, Rinehart & Winston, Inc., 1969.

SINNOTT, EDMUND W. *Cell and Psyche: The Biology of Purpose*. New York: Harper and Row, Publishers, Inc., 1961.

VOLPE, E.P. *Understanding Evolution*. Dubuque, Iowa: William C. Brown Company, 1972.

WADDINGTON, C.H. *Biology, Purpose and Ethics*. Worcester, Mass.: Clarke University Press, 1971.

WALLACE, BRUCE, and A.M. SRB. *Adaptation.* Englewood Cliffs, N.J.: Prentice-Hall, Inc., 1961.

Man and Culture

DOBZHANSKY, T. *Mankind Evolving.* New Haven, Conn.: Yale University Press, 1966.

EIBL-EIBESFELDT, I. *Ethology.* New York: Holt, Rinehart & Winston, Inc., 1970.

GOLDSCHMIDT, W. *Man's Way.* New York: Holt, Rinehart & Winston, Inc., 1967.

HOWELLS, WILLIAM. *Mankind in the Making.* Garden City, N.Y.: Doubleday & Company, Inc., 1967.

KORN, N. (ed.). *Human Evolution.* New York: Holt, Rinehart & Winston, Inc., 1973.

LESTER, D. *Comparative Psychology.* Port Washington, N.Y.: Alfred Publishing Company, Inc., 1973.

LORENZ, K. *On Aggression.* New York: Bantam Books Inc., 1970.

MONTAGU, M.F. Ashley (ed.) *Culture and the Evolution of Man.* New York: Oxford University Press, Inc., 1965.

MONTAGU, M.F. Ashley (ed.). *Culture: Man's Adaptive Dimension.* New York: Oxford University Press, Inc., 1968.

PFEIFFER, J.E. *The Emergence of Man.* New York: Harper and Row, Publishers, Inc., 1969.

REDFIELD, R. *The Primitive World and its Transformations.* Ithaca, N.Y.: Cornell University Press, 1968.

SERVICE, E.R. *The Hunters.* Englewood Cliffs, N.J.: Prentice-Hall, Inc., 1966.

Man and the Natural Environment

BRESLER, J.B. (ed.). *Environments of Man.* Reading, Mass.: Addison-Wesley Publishing Co., Inc., 1968.

COMMONER, B. *Science and Survival.* New York: The Viking Press, Inc., 1967.

DARLING, F.F., and J.P. MILTON (eds.). *Future Environments of North America.* Garden City, N.Y.: Natural History Press, 1966.

DARNELL, R.M. *Ecology and Man.* Dubuque, Iowa: William C. Brown Company, Publishers, 1973.

DASMANN, RAYMOND. *A Different Kind of Country.* New York: Macmillan Publishing Co., Inc., 1968.

DETWYLER, T.R. *Man's Impact on Environment.* New York: McGraw-Hill Book Company, 1971.

DOWDESWELL, W.H. *Animal Ecology.* New York: Harper and Row, Publishers, 1961.

EHRLICH, P.R., and A.H. EHRLICH. *Population, Resources, Environment.* San Francisco: W.H. Freeman & Co., Publishers, 1970.

ELTON, CHARLES S. *The Ecology of Invasions.* London: Methuen & Co., Ltd., 1963.

EMMEL, THOMAS C. *An Introduction to Ecology and Population Biology.* New York: W.W. Norton & Company, Inc., 1973.

GOLDSMITH, EDWARD, ROBERT ALLEN, MICHAEL ALLABY, JOHN DAVOLL, and SAM LAWRENCE. *Blueprint for Survival.* Boston: Houghton Mifflin Company, 1972.

JACOBS, JANE. *The Death and Life of Great American Cities.* New York: Vintage Books, 1961.

MARSH, G.P. *Man and Nature.* Cambridge, Mass.: Harvard University Press, 1967.

MASON, W.H., and G.W. FOLKERTS. *Environmental Problems.* Dubuque, Iowa: William C. Brown Company, Publishers, 1973.

National Academy of Sciences—National Research Council. *Resources and Man.* San Francisco: W.H. Freeman & Co., Publishers, 1969.

PADDOCK, W., and P. PADDOCK. *Famine—1975! America's Decision: Who Will Survive?* Boston: Little, Brown and Company, 1967.

PYKE, MAGNUS. *Man and Food.* New York: McGraw-Hill Book Company, 1970.

WAGNER, R.H. *Environment and Man.* New York: W.W. Norton & Company, Inc., 1971.

WALDRON, I., and R.E. RICKLEFS. *Environment and Population.* New York: Holt, Rinehart & Winston, Inc., 1973.

WOODS, B. (ed.). *Eco-solutions.* Cambridge, Mass.: Schenkman Publishing Co., Inc., 1972.

Technology and Science

CHILDE, V.G. *Man Makes Himself.* New York: Mentor Books, 1951.

DUBOS, R. *Reason Awake: Science for Man.* New York: Columbia University Press, 1970.

FERKIS, V.C. *Technological Man.* New York: Mentor Books, 1969.

GIEDION, S. *Mechanization Takes Command.* New York: Oxford University Press, Inc., 1970.

HOLTON, G. (ed.). *Science and Culture.* Boston: Houghton Mifflin Company, 1965.

KRANZBERG, MELVIN, and W.H. DAVENPORT (eds.). *Technology and Culture.* New York: Schocken Books, Inc., 1972.

KUHN, THOMAS S. *The Structure of Scientific Revolutions.* Chicago: University of Chicago Press, 1968.

MARX, L. *The Machine in the Garden.* New York: Oxford University Press, Inc., 1968.

MATSON, F.W. *The Broken Image.* Garden City, N.Y.: Anchor Books, 1966.

MUMFORD, L. *Technics and Civilization.* New York: Harcourt, Brace Jovanovich, Inc., 1963.

————. *The Pentagon of Power.* New York: Harcourt, Brace Jovanovich, Inc., 1970.

RUSSELL, BERTRAND. *The Scientific Outlook.* New York: W.W. Norton & Company, Inc., 1962.

STORER, N.W. *The Social System of Science.* New York: Holt, Rinehart & Winston, Inc., 1966.

WEINBERG, A.M. *Reflections on Big Science.* Cambridge, Mass.: M.I.T. Press, 1968.

WHITE, L., JR. *Medieval Technology and Social Change.* New York: Oxford University Press, Inc., 1966.

WHITEHEAD, ALFRED N. *Science and the Modern World.* New York: Mentor Books, 1960.

Health

ACKERKNECHT, ERWIN H. *History and Geography of the Most Important Diseases.* New York: Hafner Press, 1965.

BENARDE, MELVIN A. *Our Precarious Habitat.* New York: W.W. Norton & Company, Inc., 1970.

BOYDEN, S.V. (ed.). *The Impact of Civilization on the Biology of Man.* Toronto, Canada: University of Toronto Press, 1970.

CHASE, ALLAN. *The Biological Imperatives: Health, Politics, and Human Survival.* New York: Holt, Rinehart & Winston, Inc., 1971.

DELGADO, JOSÉ M.R. *Physical Control of the Mind.* New York: Harper and Row, Publishers, 1969.

DUBOS, RENÉ. *Mirage of Health.* Garden City, N.Y.: Anchor Books, 1959.

————. *Man Adapting.* New Haven, Conn.: Yale University Press, 1968.

FULLER, WATSON (ed.). *The Biological Revolution.* Garden City, N.Y.: Anchor Books, 1972.

HALL, EDWARD T. *The Hidden Dimension.* Garden City, N.Y.: Doubleday & Company, Inc., 1966.

KILBOURNE, EDWIN D., and W.G. SMILLIE (eds.). *Human Ecology and Public Health*. New York: Macmillan Publishing Co., Inc., 1969.

PACKARD, VANCE. *A Nation of Strangers*. New York: David McKay Co., Inc., 1972.

READ, DONALD A., and W.H. GREENE. *Health and Modern Man*. New York: Macmillan Publishing Co., Inc., 1973.

SEYLE, HANS. *The Stress of Life*. New York: McGraw-Hill Book Company, 1956.

ZINSSER, HANS. *Rats, Lice and History*. New York: Bantam Books, Inc., 1960.

The Future

BRONWELL, ARTHUR B. (ed.). *Science and Technology in the World of the Future*. New York: Wiley-Interscience, 1970.

FEINBERG, GERALD. *The Prometheus Project: Mankind's Search for Long-Range Goals*. Garden City, N.Y.: Anchor Books, 1969.

HARDIN, GARRETT. *Exploring New Ethics for Survival*. New York: The Viking Press, Inc., 1972.

HUXLEY, ALDOUS. *Brave New World*. New York: Modern Library, 1956.

KAHN, HERMAN, and ANTHONY J. WIENER. *The Year 2000*. New York: Macmillan Publishing Co., Inc., 1969.

McHALE, JOHN. *The Future of the Future*. New York: George Braziller, Inc., 1969.

POTTER, VAN RENSSELAER. *Bioethics: Bridge to the Future*. Englewood Cliffs, N.J.: Prentice-Hall, Inc., 1971.

REICH, CHARLES A. *The Greening of America*. New York: Bantam Books, Inc., 1971.

SKINNER, B.F. *Walden Two*. New York: Macmillan Publishing Co., Inc., 1962.

STENT, GUNTHER S. *The Coming of the Golden Age*. Garden City, N.Y.: Natural History Press, 1969.

TAYLOR, GORDON R. *Rethink: A Paraprimitive Solution*. London: Secker and Warburg Ltd., 1972.

TOFFLER, ALVIN. *Future Shock*. New York: Random House, Inc., 1970.
——— (ed.). *The Futurists*. New York: Random House, Inc., 1972.

TOYNBEE, ARNOLD. *Surviving the Future*. New York: Oxford University Press, Inc., 1971.

WALLIA, C.S. (ed.). *Toward Century 21*. New York: Basic Books, Inc., 1970.

General

BATES, MARSTON. *Man in Nature.* Englewood Cliffs, N.J.: Prentice-Hall, Inc., 1964.

RUSSELL, W.M.S. *Man, Nature and History.* London: Aldus Books, 1967.